Donated by:

The N.H. Jaspus Foundation, Inc.
2 Herrick Street
Merrimack, N.H. 83054

In Memory of Jordan S. Bird

LUPUS: THE BODY AGAINST ITSELF

LUPUS: THE BODY AGAINST ITSELF

Sheldon Paul Blau, M.D.
and Dodi Schultz

DOUBLEDAY & COMPANY, INC., GARDEN CITY, NEW YORK

RC
924.5
.L85
B56

76919

Library of Congress Cataloging in Publication Data

Blau, Sheldon Paul.
Lupus, the body against itself.

Includes index.
1. Lupus erythematosus, Systemic. I. Schultz,
Dodi, joint author. II. Title.
RC924.5.L85B56   616.9′78
ISBN 0-385-04562-x
Library of Congress Catalog Card Number 76-40881

To the patients,
with hope

Contents

Part One
The Puzzle

Several years ago, a nationally distributed tabloid that is inclined to elicit sales by infusing ordinary people and events with an aura of spectacle and sensation bannered its front page with a headline that read, "Half a Million Americans Have Histoplasmosis!" Which, of course, led the prospective reader to infer that the disease in question was mysterious, hitherto unknown, and a newly discovered threat to the fabric of our society if not to life itself.

The statement in the headline, as it happens, was—and still is—perfectly true. The inference is not. Histoplasmosis is a fairly widespread fungus infection of the respiratory system. A probable five hundred thousand Americans do contract it each year. It is easily diagnosed; it is typically not very serious, and it is successfully treated with a variety of antibiotic agents.

That particular tabloid has not, to our knowledge, devoted similar space and attention to lupus. The reactions of nonmedical friends and acquaintances, on learning that this book was in progress, varied from "Come again?" to "That's a tropical disease, right?" Yet lupus afflicts, at any given moment, not half a million but a probable *one million* Americans, the majority of them young women. The systemic form of lupus, with which this book is concerned, is often diagnosed only with great difficulty. It can be extremely serious, and it can sometimes kill. There is no agent or class of agents with which it can be treated with consistent and predictable success.

With the progress that has been made in defining, fighting, and preventing many of the hitherto mysterious malignant, infectious, and congenital disorders, lupus has emerged as *the* major remaining mystery of medicine.

In a sense, the picture we present in the next four chapters resembles less a complete panorama than a jigsaw puzzle created by a particularly fiendish designer, deliberately planned to frustrate and madden the solver. Some pieces are clearly linkable with others, but many are not, and it is by no means certain that all the pieces have been supplied. There are no obvious gaps to denote the missing links. The size and shape of the finished picture can only be guessed at; neither dimensions nor configuration are given. Only several sets of random clues—which will constitute the second part of this book—hint at the solution.

1. Naming the Nemesis

Many centuries ago, Hippocrates described a disease that frightened physicians and victims alike. He characterized it as an erosive, disfiguring malady, eating away at the skin and flesh of the face. We don't know what ill —or, more likely, ills—he was picturing. But in the mid-nineteenth century a number of writers bestowed the name "lupus" (Latin for "wolf") upon what they thought he had described: an affliction causing the sort of damage that might result from the bite of a ravenous wolf. They, too, were probably denoting a number of different diseases.

Foremost among them was one that came to be called *lupus vulgaris*; it is now known, much more accurately, as cutaneous tuberculosis, and it no longer causes the tissue devastation it once did, for the same reason that other kinds of tuberculosis are no longer the threats they once were: the cause of tuberculosis, whatever the parts of the body it attacks, is known, and there are medications that deal effectively with *Mycobacterium tuberculosis*, the tuberculosis bacillus.

By the 1840s, with greater understanding of infectious maladies as opposed to those that were not communicable, the term *lupus erythematosus* (LE)—"lupus characterized by redness"—began to be used to differentiate this noncontagious entity from other disorders frequently affecting facial skin, and a salient characteristic of the lupus rash was noted: a "butterfly" configuration, arching over the bridge of the nose and winging outward and downward over the cheeks on either side.

Still, it was not until the turn of the century that the distinguished Canadian physician Sir William Osler, then working and teaching at Johns Hopkins University in Baltimore, published a series of thoughtful papers concluding in no uncertain terms that lupus erythematosus was a systemic disorder, affecting various parts of the body—not only the skin, but the joints and internal organs as well, and sometimes not including cutaneous symptoms at all.

Over the next several decades a number of "new diseases" were described, only to be finally placed in the category that had come to be called "acute disseminated lupus erythematosus" and later "systemic" lupus erythematosus (SLE), distinguishing it from "discoid" lupus erythematosus (DLE), a form in which disc-shaped lesions appear on the skin and in which other parts of the body rarely, if ever, become involved. DLE is now considered probably a variant of what is a single disease—or perhaps a single *spectrum* of disease that manifests itself differently in different individuals.

Certainly the variety of manifestations is among the most striking features of lupus. That dermatologists, those medical specialists dealing with disorders of the skin, have in their texts and journals devoted much time and space to lupus is understandable. But even a cursory survey of medical literature over the past twenty or twenty-five years reveals that articles dealing with aspects of lupus have appeared in the publications of nearly every imaginable specialty, subspecialty, and branch of professional health care. Journals devoted to cardiology, hematology, psychiatry, eye-ear-nose-and-throat diseases, dentistry, respiratory disease, neurology, and gastroenterology have published lengthy and learned discussions of lupus—and so have periodicals in the fields of pediatrics and pathology, of chest disease and surgery, of allergy, pharmacology, gynecology, renal disease, and environmental health.

What *kind* of disease or disorder is lupus? In whose province does it really lie?

The interest of all those myriad specialists in lupus is legitimate. In the 1940s, lupus came to be classified, along with rheumatoid arthritis and a number of other disorders of a more or less chronic nature, as a "collagen disease." Collagen is a specific protein substance that forms an important part of connective-tissue fibrils throughout the body. Because the victims are generally adults, because these are for the most part systemic rather than localized disorders, and because there is in most instances joint inflammation, they came to be accepted as the province of internal medicine in general and of rheumatology—a subspecialty of internal medicine—in particular.

With further understanding of the nature of lupus, a second group of physicians are finding themselves equally involved. All that is connective tissue is not necessarily collagen; thus, the categorization of lupus (as well as rheumatoid arthritis) as a *connective-tissue disorder* is fast gaining favor. And as sophisticated technology has offered more insight into what lupus is, another medical specialty is also finding it a special and absorbing challenge.

That specialty is *immunology*. Related to such generally familiar words as *immunity* and *immunization*, the term suggests the study of infectious disease and the development of immunity thereto. That is indeed part of immunology's concern, but only a part. It encompasses the entire spectrum of the body's responses to provoking agents, as a class termed *antigens*—including allergens as well as infection-causing organisms such as bacteria and viruses. Such responses very frequently include inflammation of one sort or another, inflammation that is, essentially, a signal that an antigen-antibody reaction is taking place, a marshalling of the body's defenses (whether generally or locally) against the foreign intrusion.

Sometimes, when an individual has developed immunity—as by vaccination—against a particular disease-causing antigen, there is no consciousness of the threat. Sometimes, if such a mechanism has not been developed—if, for example, an individual's upper respiratory passages are attacked by one of the more than one hundred known rhinoviruses, the organisms responsible for most cases of the common cold—the raging antigen-antibody battle and its accompanying inflammation are all too evident. Still, the conflict is relatively brief. Whether the infection lasts days, weeks, or months, the battle is at last resolved one way or the other.

Lupus is different. While it may display all the characteristics of inflammatory processes found in infections, it continues—or comes and goes at unpredictable intervals—as a chronic condition, succumbing to no known antibiotics or other anti-infection agents. Further, there is no known reason for the unrelenting attack. While antibodies are demonstrably active in lupus, their activity appears undirected. Or, more accurately, *mis*directed: in lupus, more dramatically than in any other connective-tissue disorder, the body appears to have marshalled its not inconsiderable defenses against its own tissues, furiously attacking and sometimes successfully destroying what are literally the fibers of its own being.

The connective-tissue disorders are also known collectively as *autoimmune disorders*—disorders manifesting self-attack, self-repulsion on the cellular level. Rheumatoid arthritis and other connective-tissue disorders can also, to an extent, be so described. But lupus is the prototype, the classic and confounding example of what is perhaps the most perplexing puzzle in medicine (not excluding the aberrant cell proliferation of the cancers): the body actively, viciously mobilized against itself.

2. The Spectrum

"Bizarre" is one appropriate adjective that has been popularly applied to lupus. Consider the following typical cases.

Cathy, age fifteen. She first went to the doctor one summer in the 1960s complaining of aching joints, especially those of her wrists and fingers. She also had a scaly rash on her ears. Her doctor had the justifiable feeling that she'd been through an individualistic reaction to rubella, which had been making the rounds that year and frequently causes a transient arthritis, more often in teenagers and adults than in small children. The rash seemed unrelated and, like many such rashes, cleared up with regular application of a corticosteroid ointment. But a year later the joint pains returned, along with a fairly low fever. There was also a reddening of Cathy's skin over her nose and cheeks. Cathy has systemic lupus.

Alison, age twenty-eight. Married and the mother of a three-year-old daughter, Alison was hospitalized for tests when she told her doctor about her joint pains, fatigue, and weight loss that had taken place over the previous six weeks. Her doctor found that she also had a fever of 105° F. (40.5° C.). In the hospital, blood tests showed that she was also dangerously anemic, her kidneys were functioning less than optimally, one eye and one lung were similarly affected, and there was measurable weakness in many of her joints. Alison has systemic lupus.

Maria, age twenty-three. Maria consulted her family doctor when she was told at a public clinic that a test for syphilis was positive—and was baffled by a subsequent report, after another blood test, that the first report was erroneous, that "these things sometimes happen." She did not know quite what to think since there was in fact no reason for her to suspect that she could possibly have contracted a venereal disease. Her doctor found that she had a low fever, that her pulse was a bit fast (often associated with fever), and that her hands were unusually pale and cold; she mentioned that she had experienced some recent shortness of breath. Maria has systemic lupus.

Georgette, age thirty-one. An alarming pair of symptoms brought Georgette to the emergency room of a large metropolitan medical center: she was having trouble breathing, and there were strange and frightening pains in her chest. A number of diagnostic procedures were immediately performed. Georgette's chest X ray showed enlargement of the heart, a highly unusual condition in so young a woman. Further tests revealed inflammation of the pericardium, the membrane around the heart, with a collection of fluid. The fluid was removed surgically, and recovery was smooth. But it may occur again, and other problems have arisen since. Georgette has systemic lupus.

We could go on for many pages. Rashes, fever, joint pains, weight loss, fatigue, heart problems, anemia, kidney and sensory malfunction, and false-positive tests for syphilis are just a few of the many signs and symptoms with which lupus might begin or to which it might progress. Among others might be sun sensitivity, pleurisy and pneumonia, hair loss, mental or emotional problems, nausea and vomiting, jaundice, and—well, almost any adverse phenomenon imaginable. Depending upon the initial complaint, systemic lupus has been (and is) not infrequently diagnosed at first as another autoimmune disorder (especially scleroderma or rheumatoid arthritis), cancer, rheumatic fever, allergy, kidney infection, phlebitis—in fact, just about everything but the common cold.

Decades ago, syphilis—because its late-stage manifestations can be so varied and affect so many different parts of the body—was known as "the great imitator." Now the bacterium responsible for that venereal disease can be easily pinpointed and, with early testing and diagnosis, the infection can be banished, so that later, more advanced stages are rarely seen; the first stage of syphilis, in which there are typically clear and unmistakable symptoms, is now usually the stage of treatment.*

In children, some forms of leukemia are also known as "great imitators." Frequently, those cases that begin with mild symptoms can emulate a number of common childhood infections and can also assume the guise of common, nonserious injury to which youngsters are generally prone.

But *lupus* is now *the* "great imitator."

The first recognized symptom in just over half of all cases of systemic lupus is mild but persistent aching in the joints; often, as in rheumatoid arthritis, the ache and stiffness are worst in the morning and may dissipate entirely later in the day. At least eight out of ten lupus patients will experience arthritis sooner or later, and about half will suffer from muscle aches as well.

Another 15 to 25 percent first visit a physician because

* The false-positive reaction to the test for syphilis, which we mentioned earlier—it can occur in some other conditions, notably acute hepatitis, as well as in lupus—is associated with the most widespread test in use. That is the VDRL, so called because it was developed by the Venereal Disease Research Laboratory of the Public Health Service; simple and inexpensive, it is usually the initial test used by both private physicians and broad screening programs. If there is reason to suspect a false-positive VDRL, a second, different type of text—caled the FTA, for Fluorescent Treponemal Antibody—may be used. In this test, serum is withdrawn and challenged with *Treponema pallidum,* the spirochete (a type of screw-shaped bacterium) responsible for syphilitic infection; a positive result, revealing the presence of active antibody to that specific organism, confirms the diagnosis of the venereal disease. (False-positive reactions to the FTA test, while not unknown, are extremely rare.)

of the puzzling skin rashes. Sometimes the rash is on the face and assumes the classic "butterfly" form. But it may be almost anywhere, and legs and arms are common sites. The rash is invariably reddish. Seven out of ten lupus victims will have a skin rash eventually.

Typically a low fever is among the patient's initial symptoms (90 percent will run fevers at one time or another). Often the patient will report weight loss along with loss of appetite, and there may also be any one or more of a variety of other complaints: persistent swollen lymph nodes, fatigue, unusual sensitivity to the sun (contrary to some published reports, a sizable number—about one third—of lupus patients, but *not* all, display this sensitivity).

Whatever the symptoms at the start of the illness—or at the time of diagnosis—compilations of past experience suggest that other signs and symptoms are very apt to occur eventually. Among these are hair loss (there is a probability of 20 to 40 percent), cardiac problems of one sort or another (30 to 50 percent), pleuritis or pleurisy (45 to 60 percent), and major kidney-function abnormalities (perhaps half).

All or none of the above, it should be added, may occur in any one patient; the foregoing figures are statistics, not individual prognoses. But they have occurred and doubtless will continue to occur. And they are, one and all, due to the inflammatory process that marks the syndrome we call lupus: inflammation that may strike anywhere in the body, at any time; inflammation that is the hallmark of the illness; inflammation that is the evidence of the continuing battle taking place below the threshold of visibil-

important

ity, the attack of the body's defense mechanisms upon its
own cells and structures.

No one yet knows what triggers or nurtures the cellular
destruction (the latter part of this book is devoted to
speculation on this mystery), *except* for this fact: in approximately 10 to 12 percent of all diagnosed lupus cases,
the appearance of the disease has followed the administration of one of a number of drugs. And, significantly,
cessation of the drug has halted the lupus—cured it, if you
will—at least after a time (treatment may be necessary).
Spontaneous lupus, not associated with a drug, is generally chronic (as with rheumatoid arthritis, there are often
"active" and "inactive" periods—and inactive periods may
last for many years, or even indefinitely). Thus, in a small
proportion of cases, the illness—though substantially the
same at the time of its appearance as the chronic, non-
drug-related cases—is clearly provoked by a specific
agent. This similarity between the two types of lupus ex-
tends to laboratory findings, which will be discussed in
the next chapter.

A number of different types of medication have been
implicated in setting off the lupus process, and they have
little or nothing in common that might provide hints to
those seeking the cause of the "naturally" occurring disease. The best documented are—in this order—
hydralazine (Apresoline), an antihypertensive; procainamide (Pronestyl), a drug given to correct certain cardiac
arrhythmias (irregularities of the heartbeat); isoniazid
(Hyzyd, Niconyl, Nydrazid), widely used in treatment of
tuberculosis; chlorpromazine (Thorazine), a major tran-
quilizer; and methyldopa (Aldomet), another antihyper-

tensive. Occasional instances have also been reported that seemed directly associated with sulfa drugs; other powerful tranquilizers; certain antibiotics, notably penicillin, streptomycin, griseofulvin (Fulvicin, Grifulvin, Grisactin), and some of the tetracyclines; and a few anticonvulsants, in particular the hydantoins—phenytoin (Dilantin) and mephenytoin (Mesantoin)—and succinimides (Celontin, Milontin, Zarontin), as well as trimethadione (Tridione) and carbamazepine (Tegretol).

As far as symptoms are concerned, these drug-induced cases do differ somewhat from idiopathic lupus.† There is the same incidence of joint symptoms, the same likelihood of chest inflammation and congestion. And, as we noted, many abnormal laboratory findings are identical. In drug-caused lupus, however, there is little or no likelihood of swollen lymph nodes, of any kidney or gastrointestinal problems, or of any emotional or mental effects (which may occur in one in four cases of the "regular" kind of lupus), and the patient is only half as likely to have fever, a rash, anemia (a finding in perhaps half of all lupus patients), or heart involvement. These cases—of lupus, "drug-induced lupus," or, if you will, "pseudolupus"—almost invariably respond to conservative treatment consisting of withdrawal of the suspected drug and tiding

† "Idiopathic" is a widely used medical term coined from two Greek words that translate literally as "private, or personal, illness." Whatever the circumstances of the original coinage, it has come to denote any condition, whether suffered by one individual or by millions, for which no definite cause can be pinpointed. The vast majority of lupus cases are of course in this category, as are most instances of epilepsy, high blood pressure, and many other ailments.

the patient over with supportive medications and other therapies until symptoms have abated.

But, in the vast majority of cases, in a possible nine hundred thousand Americans, there is no such easy answer. In the next two chapters, we take a closer look at what lupus is: what characterizes the syndrome at the cellular level, how it can be differentiated and distinguished from other ills with some similar symptoms, and what, in the light of present knowledge, constitutes treatment of the disease.

3. Singling It Out: Diagnostic Determinants

With such nebulous initial complaints as rashes, fevers, malaise, lack of appetite, and divers aches and pains, it might seem virtually impossible to arrive at a diagnosis of systemic lupus. But diagnosis, as in any condition requiring therapy, is necessary so that appropriate treatment can be instituted—and, as important, so that *in*appropriate, or even potentially harmful, measures are not taken.

Initial symptoms might seem, for example, to suggest a bacterial infection. But if the condition does *not* stem from bacterial infection, it will not be improved by the administration of antibiotics; if the patient has lupus and happens to have multiple allergies—as many lupus patients, in fact, do—and is specifically allergic to the antibiotic used, she may well become much sicker. (We've used "she" here, and will continue to do so, both to avoid repeated use of the cumbersome "he or she" and because most people with lupus—as many as nine out of ten, according to some educated estimates—are women.)

Until very recently, however, there were no established guidelines; lupus was diagnosed, or not diagnosed, on the basis of the individual physician's experience with its various manifestations. That experience, of course, might vary from quite broad to little or none. It is highly likely that a great many cases were not diagnosed at all (and perhaps still are not).

In 1971, the Diagnostic and Therapeutic Criteria Committee of the American Rheumatism Association, the organization of physicians specializing in the rheumatic and arthritic disorders, set about the task of establishing diagnostic criteria. Calling upon leading rheumatologists throughout the United States and Canada, the committee drew up a list of characteristics—symptoms and complaints, clinical observations, and laboratory findings—that had, in the experience of the reporting doctors, occurred with significant frequency in lupus patients, based upon detailed case histories. All these characteristics were then laboriously compared with findings in an equal number of rheumatoid arthritis patients and still another group, also equal in number, of patients in whom there was no suspicion of any rheumatoid disorder.

Each of these items—there were nearly sixty in all—was tested for *specificity;* that is, the likelihood of its being helpful, in combination with other factors, in differentiating systemic lupus from rheumatoid arthritis or some

other ailment. It was noted, for example, that while peripheral neuritis (inflammation of nerves outside the central nervous system) was reported in 11.4 percent of
lupus patients, it was also found in 8.2 percent of those
with rheumatoid arthritis and in 8.8 percent of the third
group of patients—and so it was obviously a rather poor
criterion upon which to base a suspicion of lupus. Pleuritis, on the other hand, was found to occur in 60.4 percent of the lupus patients but in only 8.6 percent of the
rheumatoid arthritis patients and in 9.7 percent of the
third group—making its significance in diagnosing lupus
considerably greater.

The result was presented as a set of fourteen preliminary criteria for diagnosis and classification of patients
with lupus, with the requirement that at least *four* of the
fourteen be met in order to establish diagnosis beyond
doubt. Questions have since been raised about the inclusion of some items and the exclusion of others, and we
shall comment on some of those. First the fourteen criteria (here paraphrased in some instances and including
some explanatory language):

1. The classic "butterfly" rash over the nose and cheeks,
possibly only on one side of the face.

2. Reddish raised patches, anywhere on the body, characteristic of what was classically known as "discoid" lupus
and is now considered one possible form or manifestation
of the systemic condition (the latter may or may not sub-
sequently develop). These lesions are roughly disc-
shaped, thick, and scaly; they may leave scars after
healing.

3. Raynaud's phenomenon: paling and numbness of the

fingers due to interference with circulation in the small arteries of the hands. (It is essentially identical to frostbite.)

4. Rapidly occurring, unexplained loss of scalp hair.

5. Photosensitivity: unusual skin reaction to sunlight.

6. Ulcerative sores in the mouth, nose, or throat. (Similar sores may sometimes occur in the vagina.)

7. Arthritis in one or more peripheral joints—including pain on motion, tenderness, and/or swelling—without marked deformity. (Peripheral joints include all those of the hands, arms, feet, and legs, as well as the joints of the hips, the shoulders, and the lower jaw.)

8. Finding of two or more LE cells on one occasion, or one LE cell on two different occasions. (We'll explain what an LE cell is at the end of the list.)

9. A false-positive response to the test for syphilis, persisting over a six-month period.

10. A high level of proteinuria (the presence of certain proteins in the urine, determined by laboratory tests; it may be symptomatic of a number of conditions, including a variety of urinary-system disorders, but it is always considered in conjunction with other findings).

11. Blood casts—cellular fragments of elements normally found in the blood—in a body discharge such as sputum or urine, suggesting minute foci of bleeding within the kidney or in the tiny air sacs of the lungs (again, a laboratory finding based on specimen analysis).

12. Evidence of either pleuritis (inflammation of the pleura, the membrane lining the chest cavity) or pericarditis (inflammation of the pericardium, the outer membrane surrounding the heart).

13. Either psychosis or convulsions, occurring without any obvious explanation such as ingestion of a toxic drug.

14. Either hemolytic anemia, leukopenia, or thrombocytopenia. (All of these refer to deficits in the circulating blood; they in fact cover the three main types of blood cells. Hemolytic anemia is a deficit in erythrocytes, the red blood cells, traceable to abnormally rapid destruction of those cells. Constant creation and discard, it should be noted, is normal; an individual erythrocyte generally lives for about three months. In hemolytic anemia, the red cells are being dispensed with prematurely. Leukopenia is a deficit in white cells, basically the infection-fighting elements in blood. Thrombocytopenia is a deficit in thrombocytes, or platelets, those cells responsible for triggering clot formation in case of wounds and controlling bleeding.)

Before we comment on the validity of the criteria as they have been perceived in the years since their formulation, we shall explain criterion number 8, as promised.

The year 1948 marked a milestone in rheumatology. In that year, Dr. Malcolm M. Hargraves and his colleagues at the Mayo Clinic discovered and described a new and unique phenomenon. In material isolated from the bone marrow of a lupus patient, stained in a specific manner and placed on a microscope slide, they saw a particular type of white cell called a polymorphonuclear leukocyte, its nuclear substance pushed to one side by another such cell nucleus within it—essentially, a cell devouring the nuclear material of another of its kind. This evidence of aberrant phagocytosis (a process by which white cells normally dispose of bacteria, body discards, and other cellular debris), which can now be found by blood sampling, is the LE cell—also sometimes referred to as the LE factor or the LE phenomenon.

LE cells are not found in all lupus patients; they appear, however, in perhaps 50 to 90 percent at one time or another, especially when the disease process is active (as previously noted, there is a flare-and-remission pattern in lupus). Further, they are only very rarely found in anyone who does not have lupus: the committee study found LE cells reported in fewer than four percent of the rheumatoid arthritis cases and in a mere one half of one percent of the third, nonrheumatoid patient group. (LE cells are also sometimes found in certain other conditions, notably some systemic fungal infections. And of course it is perfectly possible that these patients may have had lupus, previously unsuspected because of atypically mild symptoms.) Thus the LE-cell phenomenon, while not an absolute guarantee—either by its presence or its absence—of correct diagnosis, is a highly specific finding.

Subsequent criticism of the guidelines—which were, as we mentioned, presented by the ARA committee solely as preliminary criteria—have hinged on two points. One is that it is entirely possible for a patient to be suffering severely from lupus while evidencing, say, only one of the required four criteria. Even firm establishment of four of the criteria does not assure 100 percent certainty of correct diagnosis; a combination of criteria 7, 11, 12, and 14, for example, might under some circumstances occur in a rheumatoid arthritis patient—or in someone suffering from neither condition.

A second is that there are a number of other findings

that have been associated with lupus to a significant degree that are not included in the criteria but are, in fact, generally utilized, along with the criteria, in actual evaluations by physicians.

Antinuclear antibodies. Antibodies are defense forces developed by the body in response to antigens—factors perceived, at that primitive cellular level, as inimical, threatening, or foreign. They are highly specific. A measles vaccination—or, for that matter, the illness itself—will result in the development of antibodies only against that particular virus. Other immunizations utilizing antigenic materials, such as those for polio, rubella, and flu, work exactly the same way. These antigen-antibody reactions are, of course, extremely helpful, since they protect the body against subsequent attack by disease-causing organisms.

Since the late 1950s, there has been noted in lupus patients extremely high levels of a different class of antibodies called antinuclear antibodies (ANA)—antibodies that act not against specific disease-causing agents but indiscriminately against the nuclear material of cells. These antibodies do not penetrate living cells; rather, they apparently react to proteins, liberated from cells, that act as antigens. It is believed, in fact, that it is this sort of antibody that contributes to formation of the LE cell. It is quite possible that the inflammatory lesions of the kidneys, lymph nodes, spleen, and other sites seen in lupus are the result of the deposition at these sites of circulating antigen-antibody complexes—which might be visualized as pockets of combat activity between these two elements.

Tests for ANA have, at any rate, proved positive in

from 80 to 98 percent of lupus patients (percentages have varied with the studies reported), but in fewer than five percent of other individuals. This finding was not included in the ARA criteria, because unfortunately no such tests had been done—and the information was therefore unavailable—in nearly 60 percent of the cases considered by the committee; there were simply not enough data in that highly controlled survey to make the inclusion statistically valid.

ANAs include several types, and recent investigation suggests that finding certain of these types—and possibly subgroups of them—may be extremely significant in diagnosis. The terms DNA (deoxyribonucleic acid) and RNA (ribonucleic acid) are doubtless familiar to the reader. These are the active materials in cells, particularly in cell replication (they are released as well, of course, in cell disintegration), and it is to these substances, among others, that the ANAs react. Each is found with two different molecular structures, which are known as "double-stranded" and "single-stranded."

Double-stranded DNA is sometimes called "native" DNA, since it is a basic constituent of human cells; antibody to it is found frequently in active stages of lupus and in at least half of all lupus patients at some time, but only very rarely in other conditions. (Antibodies to single-stranded DNA have been found as often in patients with rheumatoid arthritis and other connective-tissue disorders as in those with lupus.) In 1976, Dr. M. Edward Medof and his colleagues at the University of Chicago Pritzker School of Medicine, reporting on their study of this phenomenon over a three-year period, suggested that more sophisticated testing methods may show that anti-bodies to double-stranded DNA do not occur in *any* other conditions and that this finding is uniquely specific to lupus.

Double-stranded RNA, unlike double-stranded DNA, is normally found only in trace amounts in the tissues of mammals but occurs in significant quantities in certain viruses (a fact upon which we'll comment further in a later chapter). Antibodies to double-stranded RNA have, again, been found in about half the patients with lupus but very uncommonly in other conditions.

One or another kind of ANA is found in virtually all cases of lupus, so that while a positive finding cannot rule out another disorder, a negative one can almost always rule out lupus. Thus, ANA testing is even more sensitive than searching for LE cells, although it is less specific. (We have here used the terms "sensitive" and "specific" in a particular medical sense. A *sensitive* test or procedure is one likely to reveal the condition; a *specific* finding is one likely to pinpoint the diagnosis. Since ANAs are found in the vast majority of lupus patients, while LE cells may be absent in as many as 50 percent of such pa-tients, the former finding is more useful in, for instance, screening a group of people for the possibility of lupus; it would "miss" a maximum of 20 percent of those with the condition, while LE-cell testing might miss more than half. LE cells, on the other hand, are found extremely rarely in conditions other than lupus. They therefore pro-vide more definite confirmation of the diagnosis.)

Free DNA. A corollary to the ANAs clue is a finding of free (circulating) DNA. As we've said, the antibodies do not penetrate living cells, but interact only with liberated nuclear material. High free-DNA levels, while not specifically diagnostic (for lupus or any other condition), certainly point to abnormal cell-demolition activity.

Immunoglobulins. These are the substances found in blood serum that actually contain antibodies. While the most widely mentioned, in print and elsewhere, is *gamma* globulin (sometimes for purposes of deliberate simplification), there are actually a number of such substances. There appear, by and large, to be abnormally high overall immunoglobulin levels in lupus patients, particularly during inflammatory exacerbations (in some instances *only* at those times), and the relationship with proteinuria (one of the aforementioned criteria) is statistically significant.

In the case of gamma globulin, however, some researchers have found elevated levels in a majority of lupus patients even without marked disease activity. And dermatological studies have found deposits of three particular immunoglobulins, designated IgA, IgG, and IgM, at the juncture of the upper level (epidermis) and second level (dermis) of the skin in 92 percent of rash-afflicted skin analyzed—*and* in 60 percent of tests performed on uninvolved skin. The rate for a control group was five percent. (In discoid lupus that has not progressed to the systemic type, this deposition does *not* occur in uninvolved skin.)

Rheumatoid factor. There is, as we've already seen, some symptomatic overlap between lupus and other connective-tissue disorders, notably rheumatoid arthritis. A procedure called a latex fixation test will reveal a blood element (it's classified as a kind of antibody and is found in gamma globulin) called the rheumatoid factor in approximately 75 to 80 percent of rheumatoid arthritis patients (though not usually during the first year of illness). The test is also positive in about one third of lupus patients; its value is thus limited, but many physicians feel it is helpful in conjunction with other findings.

Sedimentation rate. Another blood test may also sometimes be employed; this is determination of the erythrocyte sedimentation rate, often abbreviated to ESR or simply "sed rate." It measures the sinking velocity of red cells within a quantity of drawn blood—a high value suggests a tendency for the cells to clump together—and here, too, there is considerable overlap with the rheumatoid arthritis picture. The ESR is elevated in about 90 percent of patients with that disorder and also in a reported 85 to 95 percent of lupus patients. (It should be noted, though, that reported results have not been consistent: some researchers have found the ESR high only when the disease was especially active, while others have found it perfectly normal even during such periods. Further, this value may be affected by any blood-cell deficits that may be present. And elevated rates can occur, too, in many infections, not excluding the common cold.)

Serum complement. A series of at least nine proteins (that number have thus far been identified), normally present in the blood, constitute what Nobel Prize-winning bacteriologist and immunologist Paul Ehrlich christened the complement system. Many, though not all, immunological reactions are dependent upon these proteins for their successful completion: attracted by antigen-antibody complexes, the "pockets of combat activity" we mentioned earlier, these proteins move in and, acting in a cascadelike manner, provide "backup" aid for the antibodies by destroying the cell membranes of the "enemy" organisms. Thus, in lupus, complement is drawn to the areas of self-destructive activity—and, because the total amount of complement in the body at any given moment is finite, there will be lower-than-normal levels circulating in the blood at such times, and a low serum-complement level is indicative of active disease. For that reason, determination of the level is helpful not only in diagnosis but in treatment as well, and the level is often monitored during therapy; a falling value may suggest increasing disease activity even before symptoms become evident, while rising levels of serum complement are typically correlated with improvement and can thus confirm the effectiveness of medication.

We shall return to some of these diagnostic factors, along with further research findings, later. In the next chapter, we summarize the past and present treatment of lupus.

4. To Hold the Line: Trends in Treatment

As we noted in the first chapter, many misleading statements have been made in defining lupus. So it is with prognosis. For the sake of lupus patients who may be reading this book in an effort to learn more of their mysterious malady, we feel it is necessary to dispel some of that misinformation.

We have before us three widely available paperback books marketed as general medical guides for the lay person. One, first written in 1959, in its seventeenth printing (1968) does differentiate lupus from the tuberculosis of the skin formerly known by that name but goes on to state that lupus is "a rare collagen disease that . . . is a chronic, progressive, usually fatal disorder." A second, written in 1962, terms lupus a "disease of the skin" that may be "associated with disease of internal organs, and death can result." The third book, with a 1966 copyright date, talks of a disease marked by "red, scaly patches" and warns that "infusion into the joints" may lead to "toxic effects" that "may be extreme, sometimes fatal."

As the reader who has been with us this far must realize, much of what is proclaimed by these three authors is nonsense. Lupus is neither rare (a possible million victims in the United States alone) nor (except for uncomplicated discoid lupus) a "disease of the skin." There is no known toxin involved. There may or may not be involvement of the skin—or, for that matter, the joints or any internal organs—although the skin is involved in 70 percent of all cases and the joints in 80 percent.

As to fatality: Involvement of the joints, contrary to the third quotation, has in no case been a cause of death. While lupus is often chronic, it is not necessarily progressive, and it is most emphatically *not* "usually fatal." The statement that "death can result" and that, when it does, it is associated with disease of internal organs, is accurate so far as it goes; its implication that death is usually or probably inevitable under such circumstances is *not* accurate. It might have been, forty or fifty years ago; it isn't now. (A great deal has transpired in the interim. In the 1930s, not only was systemic lupus usually fatal but every summer brought renewed threat of epidemic polio, appendicitis was a not infrequent killer, and the treatment of double pneumonia consisted of prayer and waiting for the crisis to pass.) By conservative estimates, the chance of survival of a lupus patient for at least ten years after diagnosis is 75 percent or more—possibly 90 percent, based on one very large recent study.

Despite the vast progress that has been made, however,

medicine remains at a distinct disadvantage in treating lupus. There are a number of reasons; we've alluded to most of them earlier, but it might be well to summarize them here.

First—and certainly foremost—the cause is unknown. As we shall see, many possible etiologies have been postulated. But none has been proved. And no present drugs known to be effective against those theoretical culprits—antibiotics against certain infectious organisms, antihistamines to stave off allergic reactions—have any effect in lupus.

Second, even its symptoms are unpredictable and frequently unexpected. Leaving infections and common allergies aside, the manifestations of most disorders, of whatever nature, can be anticipated with a reasonable degree of confidence. And usually that means that the results of therapy and nontherapy can be anticipated as well. Severe narrowing of the coronary arteries will, if uncorrected, lead eventually to myocardial infarction. Untreated diabetes mellitus will lead to coma and death. Epilepsy uncontrolled by anticonvulsant medication will result in seizures. While the etiologies of none of these are fully understood to the last detail, the cause-and-effect pattern is clear enough to indicate specific therapy and to predict the outcome of nontreatment. Even in the various kinds of cancer, while the picture becomes more complex, therapy is directed to a specific goal and its results may be determined with some accuracy; once a focus of malignant growth has been dealt with—whether by surgery, irradiation, or drugs—the sole question is that of metastasis, spread of aberrant cells beyond the original site. (Granted, detection by current techniques is not always successful, but the object of the search is nonetheless known.)

Third, as we have pointed out, treatment of lupus is restricted to dealing with signs and symptoms, rather than causation. Equally necessary are shifts in therapeutic approach as those signs and symptoms abate, intensify, or change completely. The physician and patient must thus function, in lupus as in no other condition, as a partnership—analogous, perhaps, to a police team on foot patrol, never knowing from what source trouble may appear or what its nature may be (or even if it will occur at all) but constantly prepared to cope with any eventuality and ever aware that possible incidents may range from trivial to life-threatening.

Fourth, the course of lupus is erratic. It will not run its course like an infection, or advance inexorably like a malignancy, or pose an ever-present and unchanging threat like diabetes or another endocrine disorder. It may appear, disappear, reappear—at completely unpredictable intervals of days, months, or years—and in its reappearance may assume a wholly new and different guise.

For these reasons, lupus therapy has been and is a highly individual matter. Despite advances over the past several decades, advances that have substantially reduced the rates of disability and mortality, there are no hard-and-fast guidelines and no guarantees; each patient, essentially, presents a unique situation.

Before we come to the drugs and other therapies in current use, a comment—again, chiefly for the benefit of readers who are also patients—on general care. A number of chronic ills are, for unknown reasons, subject to exacerbation by stress of various types, both physical and emotional; among them are epilepsy, peptic ulcers, migraine, heart disease, some gum disorders, hypertension, and asthma and a number of other allergic conditions. Lupus shares this susceptibility in general, with a couple of additional exacerbating factors.

The lupus patient is generally advised to avoid situations producing great anxiety and seek prompt therapy or counsel if she finds herself in a stressful situation (obviously, what produces anxiety in various individuals will differ).* Similarly, infectious ills, injuries, and undue fatigue may produce lupus flare-ups, so that they, too, must be avoided as far as possible. These are, of course, events that any prudent individual tries to avoid; it is simply a matter of degree: general measures such as balanced diet, regular physical and dental checkups, exercising of generally recommended safety precautions, etc., are helpful. Greater-than-average time allotted for sleep, and occasional rest periods during the day, are often necessary to avoid fatigue.

* It has been increasingly recognized that the unpredictable nature of systemic lupus may itself produce a good deal of stress; that is a normal and understandable emotional reaction, and abrupt mood swings that reflect the "ups and downs" of the illness itself are not uncommon. A sympathetic, supportive physician can often help to allay these anxieties. "Self-help" groups, in which patients meet to exchange thoughts and feelings related to their illness, have also been found extremely effective; a patient wishing to contact or form such a group might query her physician, the Arthritis Foundation or the Lupus Erythematosus Foundation for further information. Patients whose sexual relationships have been complicated by extreme fatigue or arthritic pain and stiffness will find some practical advice in the authors' previous book, ARTHRITIS: Complete, Up-to-Date Facts for Patients and Their Families (Doubleday, 1974).

Extreme cold can also be an exacerbating element for some lupus patients, and an individual who has found she is one of those should, take appropriate care in winter weather; for a few patients, extreme heat may have similar effects. A significant number of lupus patients—at least one third—are extremely sensitive to the sun, which may trigger not only skin lesions but arthritic symptoms and a variety of organic problems as well. Such patients should take precautions to avoid overexposure, including protective clothing (even if a limited area is exposed, such as an arm in an open car window while driving), avoidance of sunlight during the midday hours, and awareness of deceptive refracted- and reflected-light situations that can increase exposure (sand, snow, water, glass, even sidewalks can reflect light in apparent shade—and light can also be intensified by refraction through atmospheric haze and the water of lakes or pools). Effective sunscreens should be used whenever lengthy exposure to the sun is unavoidable.†

It appears, too, that allergies occur significantly more often among lupus patients than among people in general, and for that reason patients are generally advised to avoid substances widely known to act as provoking allergens in those who are sensitive to them. Permanent hair colorings are among these substances (the warning does not apply

† Effective *physical* suncreens are opaque creams, generally containing either zinc oxide or titanium dioxide, that block the sun's rays completely. *Chemical* sunscreens filter out the most harmful of those rays; they contain a variety of active ingredients, prominently para-aminobenzoic acid (PABA), padimate, glyceryl para-aminobenzoate, and several whose generic names end in -benzone. Among products most frequently recommended are A-Fil, Block Out, Pabafilm, PreSun, Solbar, Sungard, and Uval.

to water-soluble temporary rinses or to simple light-
eners), as are many ordinary cosmetics; it is wise for the
lupus patient to rely for her lipstick, eye makeup, etc., on
one of the several reputable lines of hypoallergenic cosmetics, from which the pigments and other elements most
likely to act as allergens have been excluded.

And the lupus patient should consult her physician before taking even the most innocent-seeming over-the-
counter drug. We suggest this precaution for two reasons.
One is, again, the possibility of allergic reaction. The second is the possibility of adverse interaction with a prescribed medication; many such interactions could have
extremely detrimental results, either by exacerbation of
the disorder or by interference with the intended
beneficial effects of the prescribed medication.

Medical treatment of lupus has changed radically in
the past couple of decades. Prior to the late 1940s, there
was really no drug or group of drugs that had proved con-
sistently helpful, and therapy employed a host of substances, essentially on a hit-or-miss basis; among them
were gold (some forms of which *are* effective in rheumatoid arthritis), bismuth, liver extracts, and vitamins.

Antimalarials

Immediately after World War II, the use of an-
timalarial drugs in treatment of lupus became fairly widespread. There had actually been some experimental use of
quinine as early as the 1890s, and similar drugs had also
been reported in the 1920s as having salutary effects, particularly in clearing skin lesions. The antimalarials are

now used much less, however—partly because toxic and sometimes quite serious side effects can result from their use, partly because more predictable and more controllable drugs have been developed.

The quinine derivatives—also called chloroquines—that have been most widely used in the treatment of lupus are quinacrine (Atabrine et al.), chloroquine (Aralen et al.), amodiaquine (Camoquin et al.), and hydroxychloroquine (Plaquenil). Side effects reported over the years have been many and varied, ranging from premature graying of the hair (particularly with chloroquine) to convulsive seizures (notably with quinacrine). There is a high incidence of gastrointestinal disturbance, with severe nausea and vomiting, associated with all the drugs in the group; significant numbers of patients have also suffered spotty color changes in the skin. But the most disturbing effects have involved the eyes.

One such effect involves disturbances in vision—typically blurring when the medication is started and "halo" radiation around lights later on—due to deposits of the drug in the cornea, the transparent membrane covering the pupil at the front of the eyeball; this has been seen with all the antimalarials except quinacrine. With quinacrine, however, corneal edema (swelling due to fluid accumulation) has occurred. And corneal anesthesia may occur with any of the antimalarials; this condition, in which the ability to feel pain is deadened, could be dangerous in case of accidental injury or of overexposure to sunlight. These effects disappear after the drug has been stopped.

The second kind of eye toxicity is far more serious, because it is not reversible; even after the drug is stopped, the damage remains. It involves the retina, the area at the back of the eyeball where images are focused and from which they are relayed to the brain by the optic nerves; the damage—which occurs somewhat less frequently with hydroxychloroquine—appears to result from ultraviolet-light damage and subsequent pigment deposits. The result is gradual restriction of vision—a narrowing of the visual field that may eventually progress to near or total blindness.

Use of the antimalarials in lupus is now limited to dealing with skin lesions and arthritic manifestations. And patients taking them are advised to wear protective sunglasses, both in daylight (whether or not there appears to be strong sun) and under fluorescent lights.

Three other classes of drugs now predominate in the treatment of systemic lupus: anti-inflammatory agents, both prescription and nonprescription; corticosteroids; and immunosuppressants.

Anti-Inflammatory Agents

For mild disease, the first-choice medication is aspirin—acetylsalicylic acid; it is probably the most useful medication in the entire pharmacopoeia. Best known as an analgesic (pain reliever) and antipyretic (fever reducer), aspirin also acts effectively against inflammation—which, of course, is the essential troublemaker in lupus. (It should be noted that the other salicylates, such as salicylamide, are less effective. Acetaminophen, another over-the-counter analgesic—it is sold under various trade names, including Datril, Enderin, Tempra, Tylenol, and Valadol

—is useful in countering pain and fever but does not act against inflammation.) In cases of gastric sensitivity to plain aspirin, variations such as aspirin in buffered solution (Alka-Seltzer), time-release formulations (Cama, Measurin, et al.), or specially coated tablets (Ecotrin et al.) may be recommended.

There have also recently been introduced, specifically for treatment of rheumatoid arthritis, a number of nonsalicylate anti-inflammatories that have been shown to perform on a rough par with aspirin and to result in fewer side effects—of which the major ones are tinnitus (ringing in the ears) and the gastric sensitivity previously noted— in significant numbers of patients. These prescription products include, prominently, ibuprofen (Motrin), tolmetin (Tolectin), and fenoprofen (Nalfon). Like aspirin, they diminish pain as well as inflammation. It is possible that some of these may prove useful in lupus as well.

There are a few more powerful anti-inflammatories designed for short-term, "flare-up" use in rheumatoid arthritis and some other rheumatoid disorders limited to joint involvement; they are infrequently used in lupus. The reason for the reluctance to employ them—and for their being used only on a strictly limited, short-term basis in other conditions—is a constellation of potential side effects that may involve a number of different parts of the body; they are of course eschewed completely if such effects might exacerbate problems already present in a particular patient.

For indomethacin (Indocin), the administration limit is usually weeks or months, occasionally years; side effects may include gastrointestinal sensitivity or allergic reactions (and those allergic to aspirin are often allergic to indomethacin as well), liver toxicity, intestinal bleeding, and neurological reactions including (reversible) vision difficulties.

Even more potent, and more hazardous as well, are the butazones, phenylbutazone (Azolid, Butazolidin) and oxyphenbutazone (Oxalid, Tandearil). They are absolutely contraindicated in the presence of a number of conditions that may already afflict the lupus patient—including liver, heart, or kidney dysfunction; circulatory disorders, including hypertension; and peptic ulcer—since they are themselves capable of triggering such troubles. In fact, many of the butazones' side effects simulate lupus itself; most physicians decline ever to prescribe them for lupus patients.

Corticosteroids

These are a group of agents, sometimes popularly lumped into the single word "cortisone," resembling cortisol, a hormone produced by the cortex of the human adrenal glands. There are many natural, synthetic, and semisynthetic versions and many generic names, including cortisone itself, prednisone, prednisolone, hydrocortisone, triamcinolone, paramethasone, betamethasone, dexamethasone, fluprednisolone, and more; there are dozens of brand names. The agents vary to a great extent in price and to a lesser extent in effects and side effects.

The corticosteroids are extremely useful drugs and are without doubt responsible for much of the dramatic improvement in the outlook for lupus patients. There is no question that they have time and again saved lives—not only in lupus but in a number of other acute conditions unresponsive to other therapies or for which no specific therapies exist. In lupus, they are administered in massive doses in cases of extreme, life-threatening crisis; in low maintenance dosages on a continuing basis; and occasionally for short-term therapy of a few weeks' or months' duration.

How the corticosteroids perform is still not fully understood, but their effect, in general, is to control and suppress symptoms. They have a primary anti-inflammatory action and may inhibit the production of antibodies as well. They do, at any rate, play a central role in the therapy of lupus that has failed to respond to aspirin and similar drugs (or in a patient whose sensitivity to aspirin precludes its use).

Unfortunately, there may be a number of serious side effects, which may include slowed hair growth; slowed healing of injuries; hirsutism; osteoporosis (skeletal weakening due to loss of bone substance); cataracts; masking of symptoms not only of the chronic condition but of others, such as acute infections, as well; precipitation of diabetes mellitus; aggravation of peptic ulcer (which is generally a contraindication for steroids, as is any known active infection); facial swelling; elevated blood pressure and blood-lipid levels; and, occasionally, emotional problems and other highly individual reactions. Vaccinations cannot be given to a patient receiving steroids.

Sometimes these difficulties can be minimized or avoided by carefully regulating dosages—i.e., keeping them as low as possible—and by administering them on an alternate-day regimen, in the morning. This approach can also lessen, but not avoid entirely, another side effect of the corticosteroids: suppression of the pituitary hormone ACTH (adrenocorticotrophic hormone), the normal function of which is stimulation of cortisol production by the adrenals; this occurs because there already exists a beyond-normal supply of the adrenal hormone (or a substance biochemically equivalent). (Morning administration of the corticosteroid minimizes the effect, because ACTH production is highest between 4 and 8 A.M.; steroids taken in the evening can suppress it totally.) After withdrawal of long-duration corticosteroid therapy, there is an extended period of hormonal imbalance; a therapy course of eight weeks or more may mean a year of such imbalance, with a deficiency of the natural adrenal hormones. The normal function of cortisol is helping the system to withstand sudden, massive stress; it is secreted expressly in response to such stress. So that during corticosteroid therapy, and for at least a year thereafter, serious injury or surgery poses a distinct threat unless hormonal replacement is instituted.

The corticosteroids, in short, necessary as they are in many cases of lupus, are hardly ideal drugs. They are used only in such quantities, and for such periods, as essential, and are discontinued—by tapering, rather than by sudden cessation—as quickly as possible.

None of the systemic effects are seen with the steroid-containing creams and ointments that are used, both in lupus and in other conditions, to treat skin lesions—unless there is very extensive application, particularly with dressings that do not permit air to reach the skin.

Immunosuppressants

Over the past ten or fifteen years, still another group of agents has entered the lupus treatment picture. Like the corticosteroids, they are far from ideal, they are extremely potent substances, and they are not without significant risk of undesirable effects. Nonetheless, they have proved useful in some instances.

Trials of these drugs stemmed initially from the fact that their function is to suppress deleterious immune reactions; they are the agents employed to prevent "rejection" in organ transplants, a mechanism very similar to that which occurs in antigen-antibody reactions—and appears to be occurring in lupus. Further, they also interfere with the proliferation of cells (they are used effectively in some types of malignancies)—they are also known as cytotoxins, "cell-killers"—and it was felt that they might attack the white cells that perpetrate some of the worst destruction in lupus. Prominent among these agents are azathioprine (Imuran), cyclophosphamide (Cytoxan), and methotrexate.

Clearly, such drugs may disastrously lower the body's resistance to infection (which has often been the case with the large posttransplant dosages). They have also been known to interact dangerously with a number of other drugs, including amphotericin B (an antifungal agent), anticoagulants, insulin (which is potentiated, or made stronger, in the presence of immunosuppressants), and barbiturates. Methotrexate may also interact with alcohol, aspirin and other salicylates, some tranquilizers, and sulfa drugs. And cyclophosphamide has been implicated in a number of cases of permanent sterility.

For these reasons, some physicians are still leery of any use of immunosuppressants in lupus. Many, however, feel their cautious use is warranted in the case of life-threatening disease that is not responsive to steroids. It has been found, for example, that use of small amounts of azathioprine in combination with a corticosteroid, particularly prednisone, can sometimes lower the necessary steroid dosage—and while the combination might suggest further reduced resistance to infection, the opposite has been true: the regimen has been associated in several studies with decreased incidence of serious systemic infections.

Patients reading this should know, too, that the use of immunosuppressants in lupus is strictly experimental; these drugs are research tools only, not at this writing approved by the Food and Drug Administration as standard therapy. And because of the many risks, initial enthusiasm expressed for their potential appears to be waning rapidly.

Other Treatment

As we have pointed out, lupus is a highly unpredictable entity, striking anywhere in the body with varying degrees of severity. All the general therapeutic agents are aimed at controlling symptoms. Those efforts are in most cases successful; sometimes they are not. Complications may arise, involving one or another part of the body, that are unresponsive to corticosteroids or the other currently employed therapies. Lupus patients are, of course, susceptible to the same non-lupus-related ailments as anyone else—in the case of infections, as previously noted, perhaps more so. Continued steriod therapy may not only lower resistance to infection but may also, in some cases, precipitate other problems by encouraging or exacerbating hypertension as well as hyperlipoproteinemia (increased blood-lipid levels).

Each such problem must be handled on an individual basis as it arises. Refractory anemia, for example, may require transfusion—or splenectomy, removal of the spleen. (The spleen normally sequesters and destroys red blood cells that have served their purpose and are properly candidates for discard; anemia stemming from indiscriminate, premature red-blood-cell destruction can often be remedied by splenectomy. Removal of the organ, done in some other conditions as well, generally causes no ill effects, and the spleen's normal tasks are assumed by the liver and lymph nodes.)

Fortunately, since a number of antihypertensives and antibiotics can worsen or even trigger lupus, a vast number of alternate agents have been developed in recent years. Penicillin is generally avoided if possible, but erythromycin is a highly effective alternate. Some of the tetracyclines are photosensitizing and are thus avoided, but others are not. Fungal infections, whether local or systemic, respond well to nystatin and other fungicidal agents. Immune globulins, which are available for a number of bacterial and viral infections, may be used for prophylaxis or treatment.

Circulatory deficits stemming from blood-vessel deterioration may create problems in the affected area. Prominent among these is avascular necrosis of the hip, a disabling condition involving tissue disintegration within the joint. A decade ago, crippling would have been inevitable. Now, due to advances in orthopedic surgery as dramatic as those that have taken place in chemotherapy, the joint can be completely replaced and total mobility restored. Such surgery, seemingly the stuff of which science fiction and "bionic women" are made, is now routine at major hospitals and medical centers, and tens of thousands of such procedures have been performed. (Such surgery is of course useful not only in lupus but in rheumatoid arthritis and other conditions as well.)

How many lupus patients may develop an unusual condition called *Sjögren's syndrome* is not known, but the incidence is fairly low, certainly under five percent (it is much higher, at least 10 percent and possibly over 30 percent, in rheumatoid arthritis). Sjögren's is characterized by dryness due to dysfunction of various moisture-producing glands; the lacrimal (tear) and/or parotid (saliva-producing) glands are typically prominently affected. Ophthalmological testing can confirm the eye condition; special drops ("artificial tears") are used to prevent the corneal ulceration that might otherwise occur. For mouth dryness, sugarless lozenges or citrus fruits are often suggested. If the vulvovaginal lubricating glands are involved, resulting in extremely painful sexual relations, use of a water-soluble lubricant such as KY is recommended, since such agents as petroleum jelly can be absorbed and cause systemic development of fat emboli (an embolus is a plug, of any material, blocking a blood vessel and thus preventing normal circulation).

By far the most critical threat in lupus is kidney dysfunction. Continuing antigen-antibody-complex deposits in the glomeruli, the minuscule tufts that constitute the kidney's filtering apparatus, can progress to total necrosis (disintegration of tissues) in that vital area, with the result that waste materials remain circulating in the bloodstream. Untreated uremia, the technical term for this condition, leads inevitably to increasing physical and mental dysfunction and eventual death.

There is thus constant monitoring of kidney function of lupus patients. While the various diagnostic analyses of urine mentioned earlier are helpful in this regard, glomerular deterioration is not necessarily well correlated with abnormalities in the urine itself. Far more specific is exploration of the creatinine clearance rate. Creatinine is the end-product of the action of creatine, a substance formed in the liver and necessary to voluntary-muscle contraction; creatinine, created by enzyme conversion in the muscle, is a waste product of that activity and is normally excreted in the urine. A high blood-creatinine level, indicative of a low clearance rate, suggests serious kidney dysfunction. BUN—blood-urea-nitrogen—elevation, while also hinting of kidney hypofunction, is less specific. Elevated BUN may be caused by renal disease, but it may occur temporarily as a result of other conditions, and test values may also be high following administration of certain drugs (which may actually raise the levels *or* may interfere with the testing itself).

Development of kidney dysfunction, while occasionally rapid, more typically takes place gradually over a period of months or years, and in most cases does not progress to a critical stage; many lupus patients continue to function quite well with varying degrees of renal insufficiency. But if kidney deterioration does reach that life-threatening stage and fails to respond to medication, there are only two alternatives. They are hemodialysis—periodically filtering the patient's blood through a mechanical device, an "external kidney," that performs the purification—or kidney transplant. Dialysis is still an extremely expensive, not to say tedious, procedure. Kidney transplant requires a serologically compatible donor; the five-year survival rate for patients who have had kidney transplants is approximately 90 percent when the source of the new organ is an identical twin, but drops to 50 percent when the donor is a sibling (fraternal twins are genetically no more closely related than nontwin siblings) and only 25 to 30 percent when the donor is unrelated to the recipient— although these figures are continually improving.

It is chiefly for this reason, which represents the major threat in lupus, that early control—the word "cure" cannot yet realistically be used—is so vital. And it is this ever-present threat that has spurred the intensive search for the *cause*, the factor that sets the malevolent process that is lupus in motion.

Part Two
The Clues

A number of mysterious ailments of the past, typically multisymptomatic ills, have provoked speculation as to cause and cure. It should be noted that determination of the first has almost invariably preceded the second. Exceptions have been purely fortuitous, such as the ancient Chinese predilection for tea drinking on the premise that the beverage was of divine inspiration and promoted well-being by encouraging a continuing internal harmony. In fact, boiling the water used to make the tea probably prevented a great many serious afflictions acquired by imbibing water directly from streams of doubtful purity. But, by and large, discovery of the identity of a disease-causing agent or circumstance has ultimately led to successful efforts to prevent or cure the affliction.

Earlier, we mentioned syphilis; it is an excellent example. At its various stages, symptoms of syphilis may include skin lesions of various types, heart and circulatory
malfunctions, ulcerations of the respiratory tract, arthritis,
severe muscle pains, extensive hair loss, deterioration of
the central nervous system, blindness, skeletal deformi-
ties, and psychosis.

Although syphilis had probably been observed in one
form or another throughout recorded history (some of its
manifestations were probably included in the biblical
"leprosy"), it was first recognized as a single disease entity in the late fifteenth century. Naturally, there was immediate pronouncement as to the cause—which was, the
Holy Roman Emperor Maximilian declared in 1495,
clearly divine reprisal for blasphemy, hence its designation, in that era of holier-than-the-next-nation rivalries, as
"the French disease," "the Spanish disease," "the Portu-
guese disease," "the German disease," "the disease of the
Turks," etc. (Incidentally, the French—when they were
not calling it "the Italian disease"—came to refer to syphilis as "the pox" and specifically the "great" pox, as compared with the other dreaded epidemic ill prevalent at
that time. Which is how smallpox got its name.) Subsequent theories included astrologically plotted planetary
transits (a conjunction of Mars and Saturn was particularly suspect) and atmospheric phenomena, including
both extreme humidity and severe drought.

It was not until the first decade of the twentieth century that the spirochete responsible for syphilis was discovered, although the fact that the disease was clearly
contagious, and the mode of transmission, had been es-

tablished in the interim. Specifics against syphilis, notably
an arsenic compound called Salvarsan, were soon introduced. Such drugs, despite their many and serious side
effects, remained in use until the 1940s, when the effectiveness of penicillin was unarguably demonstrated.*

While lupus has been generally recognized as a disease
entity, some still feel that it may represent a spectrum of
diseases. No mode of either acquisition or transmission is
known. No pathogen or other villain has been identified.

But there are clues—and tentative theories. Since this is
the twentieth century and not the fifteenth, the specula-
tions involve neither divine retribution, planetary vibra-
tions, nor climatic events (although the possibility of
other environmental factors can't be, and hasn't been, excluded). In the following five chapters, we single out the
most provocative observations and what may be the most
promising lines of current medical research. Which may,
we should add, seem primitive, naïve, or plainly mis-
guided when—a decade, a century, or more from now—the
answer becomes evident.

* Readers interested in exploring further the intriguing medical
and social history of venereal disease will find Theodor Rosebury's
Microbes and Morals (Ballantine, 1973) both entertaining and informative.

5. Sex Discrimination

The demographics of lupus cannot be ignored. There is a rheumatoid condition, gout, that singles out the male sex. And there are many congenital conditions—color blindness and hemophilia are certainly the best known, but there are quite a few others—that, because of a mechanism called X-linked recessive inheritance, afflict a marked preponderance of males. But lupus is, in this regard, unique: in no other known disease or disorder are such an overwhelming majority of the victims female. (We have ignored obvious exceptions specifically involving the reproductive system of one sex or the other.)

Estimates differ as to the extent of the disproportion. Several studies of large populations in recent years, however, have suggested a disparity greater than earlier impressions; it now appears that at least 82 percent, and possibly over 90 percent, of lupus victims are women.

Further, there is a distinct preference for what are generally referred to as the "child-bearing" years, the years between menarche and menopause. Although lupus has been diagnosed in both small children and senior citizens, the concentration of cases is from the teens to the forties, with a mean onset age of about twenty-nine or thirty. After the age of about fifty-five, the gender balance equalizes; as many cases of lupus are found in older men as in older women. And the mean age of diagnosis in men is much higher than in women—fifty-one years.

Essentially, then, there is a dual phenomenon: a preference for the female of the species and a concentration on her reproductive period.

The immediately evident question: Has lupus any association with estrogens, the hormones produced chiefly by females and produced in greatest quantity during this span of years? The quantity produced declines after menopause—and it is then, as we've noted, that lupus's sex discrimination tapers off as well.

It has long been postulated that the female hormones play a protective role in certain other conditions. These include both ailments that afflict a vastly greater number of men—coronary heart disease, for example—and others, including breast cancer, that strike postmenopausal women much more frequently than younger ones. Precisely the reverse pattern prevails in lupus.

Estrogen deficiencies certainly do not *cause* either heart attacks or malignancies. But these hormones *may*, as we've said, play some *protective* role. One might then ask if, in lupus, the reverse situation obtains: if perhaps androgens, the male hormones, play some part in protecting *males*. The vast majority of women, of course, are never struck by lupus. So that two corollary questions might be whether unusually *high* levels of estrogen are secreted by women who have lupus, and lower-than-normal androgen levels by male lupus patients. It must be added that androgen therapy has been tried in both male and female patients—to no avail. (It must also be pointed out, though, that "deficiencies" are not always what they seem. Vitamin "deficiencies" are known sometimes to stem from inability to absorb certain food elements. Many cases of diabetes mellitus are due not to nonproduction of insulin but to apparent inability to utilize the insulin normally.)

As this is written, there is presently underway a new study, under a grant from the Lupus Erythematosus Foundation in New York, investigating the role of female sex hormones in lupus patients. This study is especially concentrating upon the metabolism of estrogens within the body.

In 1969, an interesting report in this connection was published; it detailed the case histories of three male lupus patients who were, coincidentally (or not), also victims of a little known but not uncommon condition called Klinefelter's syndrome. The normal male's cells contain two sex chromosomes, one X and one Y. Klinefelter's is a congenital condition, occurring once in every five hundred to one thousand males (estimates vary), involving an abnormal chromosomal pattern; the cells of a male with this condition carry an extra X chromosome (it is not hereditary, but the result of conceptual accident), hence his sex-chromosome designation is XXY. Klinefelter's is characterized by, among other things, a deficit in male hormones (and is treated, generally at puberty, by administration of androgens).

On the other hand, an entirely different theory regarding the sex imbalance has been put forth in some quarters: that lupus *would* strike equal numbers of men and women among those susceptible to it (presuming hereditary susceptibility, a question we take up in the next chapter), but that an inordinate number of males in that category simply do not survive long enough to contract the condition. Many of those incipient victims, it is postulated, either succumb during gestation—i.e., are miscarried or stillborn—or, for one reason or another, do not survive childhood.

One investigator pursued this question by seeking out the living siblings of a series of almost two hundred lupus patients, managing to contact 580. While he did not find a significant preponderance of females among the siblings in general, he did find such a preponderance among those siblings born immediately before, or immediately after, the lupus patients. And there had *not* been an extraordinary number of infant and childhood deaths among the patients' brothers. His conclusion: there had possibly been some factor in their mothers' lives (or environments) at that time that had a fatal effect upon male fetuses, while the same factor had had a different impact upon female fetuses—not causing any immediate difficulties but leading to the development of lupus later in life.

Some food for further thought along hormonal lines, in any case, might be found in some of the data regarding pregnancy and lupus. This subject has been investigated by a great many researchers, since it has touched the lives of so many lupus patients.

Children born to lupus patients display no higher incidence of serious congenital problems, birth defects, etc., than children born to anyone else. There *have* been, however, a much lower proportion of children-to-be actually carried to term. About eight percent of all pregnancies, it is estimated, end in spontaneous abortion or, as it is popularly termed, miscarriage; the rate in lupus patients, according to various studies, has run as high as 30 percent, typically from 17 to 24 percent. Further, about one in four babies born to lupus patients arrives prematurely —compared, again, to an overall rate of about eight percent.

As to the effect of pregnancy on the patient herself, conclusions of various reports have differed. Most, however, have concluded that chances for remission, worsening of the condition, or no change at all are not markedly affected by the pregnancy itself (although there appears a greater likelihood of flare-up during the first trimester and to some extent during the second). But there is a significant possibility of serious worsening of the lupus *following* pregnancy, when production of progesterone, increased relative to estrogen during pregnancy, slackens (and many physicians warn patients against becoming pregnant unless there has already been a lengthy remission). The probability for severe postpartum illness is especially great in a patient who has already suffered cardiac or kidney involvement.*

* A note for patients, on contraceptive measures. Oral contraceptives—which are combinations of estrogens and one form or another of progestin, a synthetic substance resembling progesterone—have precipitated circulatory and vascular problems in a significant number of women and are especially likely to do so in lupus patients; for that reason, they are contraindicated. IUDs pose in all women some risk of perforation or pelvic infection; that risk rises, for reasons that are not fully understood, to a perilous 50 per cent in lupus. For that reason, the diaphragm is generally recommended for lupus patients who wish, or are advised, to avoid pregnancy.

Two other recently developed contraceptive methods may also hold promise. One is a device called Progestasert, a uterine insert first marketed in 1976 that, unlike the usual IUD, prevents pregnancy not by mechanical irritation (it is made of soft plastic) but by release of small amounts of progesterone over a year's time; the substance acts only locally and does not affect systemic hormone balances.

The second might be called a modern variation of the classical —and ineffective—"rhythm" method; it is a device that measures the viscosity of cervical mucus, a factor that varies more predictably during the ovulatory cycle than temperature, and can thus indicate "safe" and "unsafe" periods more reliably. It is expected to be generally available by 1977 or 1978.

6. Family Affairs

A great deal of speculation has centered about the possible role of heredity in lupus. Clearly, there is not a direct mode of inheritance as there is in a number of traits ranging from blood type, eye color, and dwarfism to disorders such as cystic fibrosis, color blindness, and sickle-cell anemia. But there are many ailments in which a predisposition or susceptibility is known or strongly suspected to be inherited, although the mechanism is not wholly understood; among them are diabetes mellitus, migraine, psoriasis, epilepsy, and most allergies.

One avenue of investigation has been that of examining and testing close relatives of lupus patients in search of either other cases of lupus or characteristics associated with lupus and/or other rheumatic disorders. The search has proved fruitful: there have been many reports detailing just such findings, far too many to attribute them to mere coincidence.

Typically, these studies have turned up not especially large numbers of lupus sufferers but constellations of unusual findings. One such study, for example, involved a lupus patient with an unusually large group of relatives available for study. The patient's mother, although she did not have lupus, did evidence hyperimmunoglobulinemia (as we noted in Chapter 3, a characteristic finding in lupus). Additionally, one of the patient's four sisters had diagnosed systemic lupus, and two other sisters and a brother hyperimmunoglobulinemia. There were no abnormal findings in the patient's two young daughters, but among nieces and nephews (at the time of the report, most were under the age of twelve years) were one girl with lupus, one girl with rheumatoid factor, a boy with both rheumatoid factor and hyperimmunoglobulinemia, and five more boys and a girl with hyperimmunoglobulinemia. All of these findings are far in excess of random determinations in the general population.

Similarly, a Scandinavian researcher delved into the families of 72 lupus patients, comparing close blood relatives with relations by marriage, who served as controls. In a 1972 report, the investigator recorded that the close blood relatives exhibited important lupus-associated features. These included 22 percent of the patients' daughters and 4.5 percent of their sons (but none of the offspring of the control group), as well as 24 percent of their sisters (the control-group rate was 9 percent). Again, the sex bias we discussed in the previous chapter is evident.

There have been quite a few reports of identical (monozygotic, originating from a single fertilized egg cell) twins with lupus—a significant point, because identical twins are identical not merely in appearance but in genetic inheritance. An interesting sidelight, related to the speculation on the role of hormones discussed in Chapter 5, emerged in a case reported in 1975 in the *Journal of the American Rheumatism Association*, a case involving a lupus patient whose identical twin had *not* developed the condition. The women were forty-four at the time of the report. One had had lupus since the age of thirty-seven, and her tests for LE cells and antinuclear antibodies were positive; her sister's were negative. *Both*, however, displayed the classic false-positive reaction to the VDRL test for syphilis (the more accurate FTA test was negative for both), and both had unusually high immunoglobulin levels, in particular IgM. But the factor that struck the investigators was that the twin who did not have lupus had been successfully treated for ovarian cancer at the age of twenty-one; her treatment had involved oophorectomy and hysterectomy—removal of both ovaries and uterus (she had not been given hormone-replacement therapy). The report's tentative conclusion: it is possible that the susceptibility to lupus is inherited *and* that the female hormones play a "permissive" role (or negate the "protective" role of androgens), "allowing" some environmental agent to cause lupus or to trigger its development.

The most comprehensive twin study in connection with lupus was reported at a 1975 ARA meeting; twelve sets of twins in which one or both had lupus were included. Extensive blood tests and physical examinations were performed, as well as chromosomal analyses designed to establish the type of twinship in each pair beyond doubt.

Seven sets of twins were proved to be identical. In four of these pairs, both twins were lupus patients; in five, antinuclear antibodies were found in both twins; in six, both twins had hyperglobulinemia. Three of the twelve sets of twins were proved to be dizygotic ("two-egg"), or fraternal, twins—no more closely related genetically than siblings of different ages. Among these fraternal twins, only one of each pair had lupus; and among the unaffected twins, blood tests revealed abnormalities in only one.

Another aspect of the heredity hypothesis is the observation, which has been made by many, that the incidence of lupus appears to be increasing. This is a somewhat speculative area. As with other disorders presenting difficulties in definition and diagnosis, technological advance and the development of highly sophisticated diagnostic techniques have made possible far more accurate case-finding. The discovery of the LE-cell phenomenon has certainly been a key factor, and so have modern methods of serological analysis. It is thus very hard to determine whether a remarkable increase in reported cases reflects actual rising incidence, improvements in diagnosis, or simply broader reporting of cases due to heightened interest in the disorder. Certainly the last two elements are involved as far as lupus is concerned, and possibly all three.

If the statistics indeed reflect true rising incidence, some observers feel that it might possibly tend to support the heredity theory. Certain other disorders in which the condition, or a predisposition, is without question inherited have in fact been increasing. The reason: improvements in therapy that have prolonged life and permitted greater opportunity for victims to pass on the genetic factors involved. A prominent example is diabetes mellitus. Prior to the advent of insulin therapy in the 1920s, the vast majority of insulin-dependent diabetics did not survive long enough to produce any significant number of offspring. Since that time, such individuals have grown to adulthood, many have become parents, and the incidence of diabetes mellitus has in fact risen dramatically. Successful medical management of conditions such as cystic fibrosis (which is directly heritable) suggests that statistics will shortly reflect rising incidence there as well. Similarly, there have been marked advances in the treatment of lupus over the past two and one half decades, with vast improvement in prognosis and life expectancy. The majority of lupus patients now live active, productive lives—and many have become parents.

The role of enzymes in familial disorders has received increasing attention in recent years. It has now been established that in several such congenital disorders—some evident immediately at birth, others not displaying signs or symptoms until months or even years thereafter—there are deficiencies in specific enzymes involved in the metabolism of certain lipids and proteins; these conditions include phenylketonuria, Tay-Sachs disease, Fabry's disease, and others.

No such clear-cut finding has been made in lupus. But there has been one recently reported study of an enzyme called acetyl transferase, which is produced by the liver and is involved in a number of biochemical processes including metabolism of certain kinds of drugs. Abnormally low activity of the enzyme can be revealed by determining the rate of breakdown of such drugs within the body: the longer the drug persists, the lower the level of activity. The study employed a series of patients in whom drug-induced lupus had been diagnosed, in this case induced by the antituberculosis drug isoniazid. These patients were compared with a like number of tuberculosis patients on isoniazid therapy who had evidenced no signs or symptoms of lupus and served as controls. Half the control group were found to have somewhat lower-than-normal acetyl-transferase activity. *All* the patients in the lupus group evidenced a severe reduction in enzyme activity. This finding suggests that naturally occurring lupus may be no different from drug-induced lupus—i.e., both may involve a constitutional metabolic abnormality.

Which brings us to the final facet of the heredity question: mode of inheritance. All of the other hereditary disorders we have mentioned are recessive, whether X-linked or autosomal—a mechanism that simply would not fit the demographic facts of lupus. Those terms may, for some readers, require a bit of explanation, which will necessarily be brief and somewhat oversimplified.*

Each human zygote, or fertilized egg cell, contains 23 pairs of chromosomes, half contributed by the ovum (egg cell) and half by the sperm uniting with that ovum. One pair are the sex chromosomes. Each of a normal female's body cells has two X chromosomes (she is designated XX), and she can contribute only an X to her offspring; a normal male has one X and one Y (XY), and his sperm may carry either. The other 22 pairs of chromosomes are called autosomes.

All the chromosomes carry genes, the units in which

---

* Readers wishing to explore the subject in depth will find it thoroughly and lucidly covered by Amram Scheinfeld in *Heredity in Humans* (Lippincott, 1972).

hereditary information is encoded, and each trait has its fixed place, technically termed its locus, on a particular chromosome. The emergent trait in a particular individual depends upon the combined information contributed by the genes at corresponding loci on each pair. If information is the same at corresponding loci, the individual is said to be homozygous for the trait in question; if not, the individual is heterozygous for that trait.

A familiar illustration is eye color. An individual who has received genes for blue eyes from both parents is homozygous for eye color and is blue-eyed; similarly, genes for dark eyes from both parents will mean the individual is homozygous for eye color and has dark eyes. Each can pass on only like information to his or her offspring. But someone whose eye-color inheritance is heterozygous—i.e., there is opposite information at the corresponding loci on the particular pair of chromosomes involved—will *not* have eyes of some neutral hue; he or she will have dark eyes. That is because, for certain traits, one message is dominant and will prevail over the opposite, which is termed recessive; eye color is one such trait, and the gene for dark eyes is dominant. An individual heterozygous for a particular trait may pass on *either* piece of genetic information to his or her offspring.†

† Lest readers whose eyes appear neither clearly blue nor clearly dark feel slighted, further comment is perhaps in order. All coloring in the body, of the eyes as well as the skin and hair, depends chiefly upon a brownish pigment called melanin. Apparent color of the iris, which is to a degree translucent, results from the amount and distribution of pigment combined with reflective phenomena, and individual eye structure is also a factor. A small amount of pigment, concentrated in the deepest layer of the iris, will be perceived as

The "odds" for a particular autosomal trait that behaves in this dominant-recessive manner may be easily calculated, and they are the same for all such traits. We can designate the homozygous individual either "DD" (in the case of eye color, dark-eyed) or "RR" (light-eyed), the heterozygous individual "DR" (dark-eyed). Simply noting the various possible combinations reveals the probabilities:

Parental Genes	Possible Combinations	"Odds" for Offspring
DD+RR	DR only	All heterozygous
DD+DR	DD, DD, DR, DR	50% heterozygous, 50% dominant-homozygous
RR+DR	RR, RR, DR, DR	50% heterozygous, 50% recessive-homozygous
DR+DR	DD, DR, DR, RR	50% heterozygous, 25% dominant-homozygous, 25% recessive-homozygous

blue. While the genetic mechanism is not fully understood, scattered depositions of pigment in upper layers of the iris apparently produce the hues we perceive as gray, green, hazel, etc.—essentially variants of the recessive trait. It should also be noted that the likelihood of two light-eyed persons producing a light-eyed child is actually not 100 percent but an estimated 98 percent; uncommonly, the normally dominant gene for dark eyes seems for unknown reasons to behave in a recessive manner.

Dark eye color is dominant to light not only in humans but in most other mammals as well. The presumed reason is that the heavier pigment concentration in the iris protects the retina from excessive light and also serves to concentrate more efficiently the light rays passing through the pupil.

If the recessive trait in question is not light eyes but a disorder, it will be immediately apparent, from the second and fourth situations, how two healthy individuals' genes might combine to produce a child with either the recessive gene or the disorder itself. (It must be noted that the "odds" in the last column prevail anew for each child, just as the outcome of a second flip of a coin is not determined by the outcome of the first.) With a few exceptions, autosomal hereditary disorders *are* recessive; all the well-known ones are, including cystic fibrosis, phenylketonuria (PKU), Tay-Sachs disease, albinism, and the hereditary anemias. In some such disorders, including sickle-cell anemia, the heterozygous individual may display the condition to an extent but in very mild form.

There is no preference displayed for either sex in traits or conditions that follow this straightforward dominant-recessive mode of inheritance. Hence, if it prevails in lupus, there must be some other factor or factors involved, certainly having to do with sex differences per se, and very possibly—as discussed earlier in this chapter and in Chapter 5—with sex hormones.

The other technical term we used earlier is "X-linked." There are quite a few traits, virtually all disorders of one sort or another, dependent upon genes carried on the X chromosome. They are practically all recessive, specifically to a "normal" gene on another X chromosome. Thus, since the normal male is XY and has no "counteracting" gene, the vast majority of those affected by these conditions are males; among X-linked recessive disorders that display this pattern are hemophilia, Fabry's disease, classic red-green color blindness, and vasopressin-resistant

diabetes insipidus. Again, as with the autosomal reces-
sives, heterozygous "carriers"—here invariably females—
may evidence minimal symptoms of the condition.

Clearly, lupus cannot be of X-linked recessive inheritance. Is there such a thing as X-linked *dominant* inheritance? Yes, there is; it is extremely rare, but a few such
conditions have been documented. (None are major disorders. One, for example, involves discoloration of the
teeth due to defective enamel.) Following the dominant-
recessive pattern, there would be a fifty-fifty chance for
an afflicted woman to transmit the gene to her offspring
of either sex; an afflicted male would transmit it to all of
his daughters but to none of his sons.

Two theories relating to possible X-linked dominant inheritance of lupus have been expressed. One is that such
a pattern does prevail but that the gene that might otherwise precipitate the development of lupus in male
offspring is "countered" by certain other factors—perhaps
by a gene on the normal Y chromosome, perhaps by the
presence of a preponderance of androgens as suggested in
Chapter 5.

A second theory postulates a constellation of genetic
factors: the X-linked dominant (possibly involving more
than one gene) *coupled* with autosomal traits, combining
to create a congenial climate for the precipitation of lupus
by environmental factors or agents.

In the next chapter, we examine the evidence relating
to one prominent class of suspected precipitators.

7. The Viral Connection

As we have seen, people like to be able to pin down causes for ailments. It makes things, well, neater. That has, of course, been true since the dawn of history. Ills have been ascribed not only to divine displeasure, astrological events, and ill winds (as we saw in the case of syphilis), but to demons, witches, and assorted bad habits.

The culprits sought in our own century are a bit more specific. A number of microscopic organisms have been unequivocally shown to cause a host of human ills from plague to warts. The common cold can confidently be blamed on some 117 separate viruses. It follows that such agents are suspected of being behind some of the more complex maladies still frustrating medicine. Lupus is one of them.

By and large, evidence of infection—whether viral or bacterial—may be adduced in two ways. One is by isolating the agent from the patient and clearly identifying it. The second is by demonstrating the existence of antibodies to that organism, which shows evidence of either present or past activity of the agent. (Antibodies, you will recall, are produced by the body only in response to specific antigens.) Those, at least, are the recognized procedures in infections that behave according to the rules—which most infections do. But not all. Or not always: it is now known that some viruses, in particular, may behave in an extremely aberrant manner under some circumstances.

We'll return to the first of those procedures and see how the scientists have fared. Before that, let's look at the second. Have unusual numbers of antibodies to known infectious agents turned up in lupus patients?

They have—and they appear to be highly specific. As you may imagine, no such agent has been overlooked; investigators have considered, and sought to eliminate, every bacterial, fungal, protozoan, rickettsial, viral, and other kind of organism known to cause disease of any description in human beings. Only one group remains suspect: viruses. And certain types of viruses have been discounted as well.

While some viruses remain unclassified, the great majority have been categorized in various groups according to their size, structure, and other characteristics. There are, for example, the *arboviruses*—short for "arthropod-borne," reflecting the fact that they are transmitted from person to person (or from animal to person) by arthropod vectors such as ticks, mosquitoes, etc.; the ills they cause include equine encephalitis, dengue, yellow fever, and others. None of the arboviruses has been implicated in lupus.

The flu viruses—the well-known A and B strains, plus a related C strain that causes occasional mild infections—are classed as *myxoviruses,* viruses that have a particular affinity for mucous membranes (their name derives from the Greek *myxa,* "mucus"). Lupus patients have *not* been found to have higher antibody levels to these viruses than anyone else.

Likewise, several other viral categories have been exonerated; at least, no evidence has been found that points to their involvement. They include the *herpesviruses,* the ones responsible for cold sores, most canker sores, chickenpox and shingles, and a number of other conditions featuring skin lesions of one sort or another; the *poxviruses* (the smallpox virus is the most prominent member of this group); the *adenoviruses* (the first part of the word is short for "adenoids"), which circulate more or less constantly among children—causing a variety of nose, throat, and eye infections—and to which most adults have high levels of antibodies; the *enteroviruses* (normally found in human intestine), which include the polioviruses and others; and some smaller groups.

There have been conflicting reports regarding a group called *parainfluenza viruses.* There are four known strains of these viruses (characterized simply by number), typically causing simple colds in adults but far more serious respiratory ills—notably croup and bronchopneumonia—in infants. Some researchers have reported unusually high levels, in lupus patients, of antibodies to the parainfluenza viruses in general (that was true of the twin with lupus we talked about in Chapter 6—but not of her sister). One 1971 investigation reported high levels only of antibodies to parainfluenza 1; two other studies the same year found lupus patients no different from control groups in that regard but reported significantly higher levels of antibodies to parainfluenza 2. Several 1973 studies appeared to confirm the significance of parainfluenza 1. The meaning of these contradictory findings is not clear.

(It should be noted that the parainfluenza viruses are quite widespread and that, as with the adenoviruses, antibodies are found in the majority of people. Some of the reported conflicts have hinged upon the differing significance attributed to particular titers—measurements of antibody levels in the blood—by various researchers.)

Earlier, we mentioned enteroviruses. Within that category is a subgroup called *ECHO viruses*, the acronym standing for "enteric cytopathogenic human orphan" viruses; the "orphan" relates to the belief, when these viruses were first identified, that they did not cause any illnesses.* It is now known that the early supposition was untrue. While most of the ills caused by the ECHO viruses are minor, they are major agents of viral meningitis.

That is by way of introduction to the fact that there is a similar group known as *reoviruses,* the first part of the

* We do not, frankly, know what led to the "orphan" designation, but the word does conjure up a touching picture of a small, helpless, and homeless wanderer, innocently fending for itself as best it can.

word standing for "respiratory enteric orphan." They
were formerly grouped with the ECHO viruses but are
now considered a separate class. A number of studies
have recorded a significantly high percentage of lupus patients with antibodies to these viruses, in particular the
strain known as reovirus 1 (one investigation found such
antibodies in 55 percent of a group of lupus patients, in a
mere three percent of an equal number of controls).
Reoviruses have occasionally been found in association
with mild febrile ills and with bouts of mild diarrhea, but
no cause-and-effect relationship has been proved.

The alert reader may be aware that a number of major
viral diseases have not been mentioned: measles, for one;
mumps, for a second; rubella is a third. The measles and
mumps viruses have been classed as *paramyxoviruses*
(they are similar to, but larger than, the myxoviruses);
the virus that causes rubella has been tentatively placed
in this category. And it is here that the most telling data
have been reported. Quite a few of the studies of lupus
patients have found higher incidence, and higher titers as
well, of antibodies to the mumps virus; most reports have
cited the rubella virus; and *the measles virus has been
listed without exception.*

There are a number of reasons why this fact may be extremely significant. They relate both to hints that have
emerged in other research on lupus and to recent revela-
tions and hypotheses regarding two other conditions.

One point is the nature of the suspect virus(es). All
viruses are classed generally as either deoxyviruses or
riboviruses, according to whether their cores consist of
deoxyribonucleic acid (DNA) or ribonucleic acid

(RNA). Many of those we listed earlier as believed inno-
cent of any connection with lupus—including the herpesviruses, the poxviruses, and the adenoviruses—are deoxyviruses. The paramyxoviruses (as well as the reoviruses,
the parainfluenza viruses, and the myxoviruses) are riboviruses, viruses with RNA cores. As noted in Chapter 3, a
marked incidence has been found in lupus patients of antinuclear antibodies to both double-stranded DNA and
double-stranded RNA; the latter is a type common in
RNA viruses but not in mammalian tissues.

We said earlier that one traditional proof of the usual
infectious disease is isolation of a specific virus from the
patient. No clearly identified virus has been isolated in
lupus. But something very suggestive of a virus or some
form thereof *has* been found.

The first to describe such findings was Houston's Dr.
Ferenc Györkey, who in the late 1960s reported isolating
material he characterized as "myxoviruslike" structures;
he and his colleagues suggested in a later report detailing
similar findings that these appeared to be "subviral structures" rather than entire viruses. It has been confirmed
that the structures consist of RNA.

Since Dr. Györkey's initial announcement, a number of
other investigators have pursued the same avenue of
research, with the same results. All have described the
structures or particles as "myxoviruslike" or "paramyx-
oviruslike." They have been found in the kidneys, skin,
white cells, nerve cells, and other tissues of lupus patients. (It is notable that at least one reported instance involved a kidney transplant. The mysterious particles had
been found in the patient's own kidneys. At the time of

surgery, the new kidney was proved virus free. One month later, biopsy of the new kidney revealed identical particles.) A few researchers have reported finding them in isolated cases of other rheumatic diseases. They have *not* been isolated from any healthy controls.

If the measles virus or another RNA virus is in fact implicated in lupus, it is certainly not via the viral mechanisms with which we are familiar.

Some have theorized that the situation might be compared to the behavior of the herpesviruses, which are known to persist after causing an initial infection and to reemerge even years later to trigger the same or other problems. The two herpes simplex viruses, for example, retire and reemerge unpredictably; type 1 causes cold sores or canker sores, type 2 genital lesions. The varicella-zoster virus initially causes chickenpox—and may reemerge years later to precipitate a case of painful shingles in the same individual. But the virus can be isolated in these later reappearances. Further, it remains communicable; some chickenpox epidemics have, in fact, started with exposure of a child to an adult with shingles. Lupus is, of course, not contagious.

It is more likely that explanation of the phenomenon— assuming the postulated viral connection does exist—lies in another direction: the etiology that has come to be known as the *slow virus*. Most of the handful of conditions traced to such a mechanism are limited to isolated exotic climes or are of decreasing epidemiological interest (parkinsonism, one of the latter, afflicts no one born after 1931, and the virus originally responsible apparently no longer exists). Two, however, are of continuing interest, particularly in connection with the research we have detailed in this chapter.

One is Dawson's encephalitis or subacute sclerosing panencephalitis, known to physicians and lay persons alike simply as SSPE. It is an illness that involves insidious, gradual deterioration of the brain, with concomitant neuromuscular, sensory, and mental disintegration; its victims are typically between the ages of five and twenty, three quarters of them boys (the reason for the gender imbalance is still unknown). There is no treatment, and death is inevitable. Thirty to fifty new U.S. cases have been reported annually in recent years; it is believed that there may be twice that number.

Early on, research in SSPE had revealed strange structures or particles in brain tissue—structures described as "myxoviruslike." Later, as suspicion of viral etiology grew, antibodies were investigated; markedly elevated titers of antimeasles antibody were found in SSPE patients. Finally, in 1970, measles virus itself was isolated from the brains of victims, and it was established that SSPE is, in fact, due to apparent reactivation of that virus—"smoldering," meanwhile, in both central-nervous-system and lymph tissues—in a child who has had measles.

Of course, most children who have had measles do not later fall victim to SSPE. (A measles vaccine was introduced in 1963, but it was not established until recently that immunization before the age of one year does not provide reliable protection. With increased public awareness of that fact, care on the part of parents and physicians to see that children are properly vaccinated, and—it is hoped—decline of measles itself, the incidence of SSPE may decline as well.) It is evident that some agent or factor must account for its selectivity, some factor that "awakens" the virus (or permits it to remain in the first place). Aside from the sex imbalance, SSPE is known to be most prevalent in the Southeast. And one major study has found a history, in a significant number of SSPE cases, of contact with a dog suffering from canine distemper—which, perhaps entirely coincidentally, is caused by an RNA virus.

The other condition in which parallels with lupus—as well as with SSPE—can be drawn is multiple sclerosis (MS).

Some 250,000 Americans are believed afflicted by multiple sclerosis. Like SSPE, it is more prevalent in one part of the country—but in the North rather than in the South (it is some forty times more common in Minnesota, for example, than in Mexico City).† Like SSPE, it affects the nervous system. Unlike SSPE, but like lupus, it is chronic

† On a world-wide basis, MS is most prevalent in two broad bands that encircle the globe both north and south; these are basically the cool temperate areas, from approximately 40° to 60° latitude. A study reported in late 1976 revealed an interesting sidelight. In that investigation, a group of British researchers explored the effects of migration to or from such areas of statistically higher "risk" upon the actual incidence of MS. The age of fifteen appears, from the results, to be a significant one. Among those emigrating from Great Britain, a "high-risk" area, to a "low-risk" locale after the age of fifteen, the incidence of MS proved no different from that prevailing in England; conversely, immigrants to Great Britain from "low-risk" parts of the world after that age are still at lower "risk." And those in the latter group whose parents had also been born in "low-risk" areas showed a still lower MS incidence—strongly suggesting the possibility of genetic as well as environmental factors, at least in susceptibility.

and may have no particular effect on life expectancy. And there are a number of other similarities to lupus, as well.

Like lupus, MS typically strikes between the ages of fifteen and forty (although there is no particular sex preference). The primary kind of lesion is demyelinization (disintegration of the sheath surrounding nerves and its replacement by scar tissue), a phenomenon that, while not predominant, is sometimes seen in lupus. As in lupus: familial "clusters" have been reported; the condition may be aggravated by extremes of heat or cold; unusually high levels of antibodies to measles, as well as some other viruses, have been found in MS patients; a relapse-and-remission pattern is frequent; there has been some therapeutic success with corticosteroids (though not to the degree seen in lupus). There have, further, been at least eight cases reported in which laboratory findings suggested lupus—while the clinical picture was that of typical MS. Like lupus, MS is often referred to as an "autoimmune" disorder. (Some have tentatively wondered if some cases of MS—even, perhaps, all cases of MS—represent a special form of lupus.)

And, in late 1975, Drs. Gertrude and Werner Henle and Drs. Paul and Ursula Koldovsky of Philadelphia confirmed the existence of a "viruslike" agent in the brain and sera of MS patients. It has not been found in healthy controls.

Both SSPE and MS have been investigated primarily by neurological researchers. With the establishment of a "slow virus" etiology for the former, there is strong suspicion in neurological circles of such an etiology in MS as well.

Viruses are essentially parasitic organisms; they are dependent upon living cellular material for their survival and propagation (hence are more difficult to study than such organisms as bacteria, which can be grown in broths and other nutrients in the laboratory—while viruses require live animals, fertilized eggs, or tissue cultures). Normally, in a process called replication, a virus attaches itself to the host cell at predetermined receptor sites, penetrates the cell, and loses its outer coat, releasing nuclear material (DNA or RNA, as the case may be); it then reassembles and is released by the cell—now infectious, but also now vulnerable to the host's defense mechanisms. That is what happens in an ordinary infection. That is *not* what happens when a virus becomes a "slow" virus, reappearing years later in altered guise to set off not an acute, contagious infection but a noncontagious condition either chronic or acute.

One theory that has been put forth, specifically relating to multiple sclerosis but possibly relating to lupus as well, is that, for some reason, the host cells fail to release the virus following replication. The theory postulates that the presence of the virus stimulates the formation of antibodies but that those antibodies are unable to attack the virus, because it still remains hidden within the body's cells. Thus, the antibodies attack what is available: the cells of the host.

(It should also be mentioned that the paramyxoviruses require an enzyme, produced by the host, for activation. Thus, it has been postulated that if the required enzyme is lacking—a deficiency that has not been specifically pinpointed in any of the disorders we've mentioned—the virus might simply linger an abnormally long time within the cell, causing damage to the host cell itself.)

Dr. Charles Christian, a distinguished researcher associated with Cornell University Medical College, has pointed out that whatever the virus (if there is a virus involved), it is clear that antigens, stimulating the production of antibodies (and inflammation) evidently persist. He has suggested the possibility that the virus, persisting within the host cell, alters the cell in such a way that some constituents of the cell are no longer recognized as belonging to the host by the immune-defense mechanisms —and "become," in that sense, "foreign" antigens. That may lead, in turn, to the fight-the-foreign-substance activities that cause the inflammation seen in lupus.

It is known that genes of the "slow" viruses are capable of actually integrating themselves into the genes of human cells. Moscow's Dr. V. M. Zhdanov established in 1974 that the measles virus is capable of that sort of activity. In 1975, Dr. Zhdanov reported that he had found nuclear material derived from the genes of the measles virus in the genes of a number of lupus patients—but not, significantly, in a group of controls. Dr. Zhdanov's intriguing theory is that the virus somehow integrates its genes into the genes of the victim's cells; the genes then produce a variety of new proteins, which proceed to incorporate themselves into the host cell membranes. There they act as antigens—biochemically "fooling" the body and its defense mechanisms into viewing them as foreign matter and initiating the inflammatory process.

Any, or none, of these theories may be correct. In any case, another question remains: Why are some individ-

uals singled out? Whether the troublemaker is the measles virus or some other known or unknown agent, why
are some individuals and not others (or some families and
not others) susceptible? The explanation may lie within
the extraordinarily complex network of bodily defenses—
the immune system.

8. B Cells, T Cells, and Forbidden Clones

Certainly the most mysterious aspect of lupus is that phenomenon called autoimmunity—mobilization of the body's defense system against the body itself. Not only do lupus patients evidence higher-than-normal antibody levels against particular viruses; they also evidence antibodies that can be clearly shown to be specifically primed for battle against the body's own tissues—against the patient's own red cells, blood vessels, muscles, and other organs.

The immune system revolves especially around a subgroup of the leukocytes, or white cells, called lymphocytes. Production of these cells begins very early, in the embryonic yolk; it continues in the fetal liver; after birth, it is centered in the thymus gland and in bone marrow.

This initial activity produces, actually, immature cells called *stem cells*, essentially defenders-to-be not yet differentiated as to function. Differentiation takes place during maturation of the cells.

Some mature in the thymus and emerge as distinct entities known as T (for "thymus-dependent") cells; others mature in the bone marrow and emerge as B (for "bone-marrow-derived") cells. Both types proceed, as mature, competent lymphocytes, to their stations throughout the body: the lymph nodes, the blood, the spleen, and various tissues and ducts situated primarily in the thorax.

T cells participate prominently in cell-mediated immune responses, interacting directly with antigens. They apparently constitute the body's first line of defense against a number of microorganisms, including many bacteria and most viruses; recent studies strongly suggest that they also play a leading role in transplant rejection and in a "surveillance" system that guards against potential malignancies.

B cells give rise to plasma cells and effect antibody responses via the production of immunoglobulins. They are believed to play the major role in repelling incursions by coccal bacteria, a few of the viruses, and certain toxins.

As we have emphasized, these defenses are brought into play against specific provoking agents or antigens, which must first be encountered in order that the process be initiated. An antigen may be defined as a chemical "flag" carried by the invading cell (be it that of a bacterium, a virus, a poisonous substance, or transplanted tissue) that identifies it as not belonging, not self. What normally happens is roughly as follows. (As in Chapter 6, we have here highly simplified what is in fact an extremely complex biochemical process.)

Upon encounter with a specific antigen, the lymphocytes respond in a predetermined manner. A few cells of both types are altered, become replicating lymphoblasts, and undergo a series of divisions that produce, in the end, groups of identical "daughter cells" equipped to repel that particular antigen.

The B cells' daughters, or "effectors," are plasma cells coded to produce specific immunoglobulins. The new T cells release substances called lymphokines, chemicals that can kill or otherwise disable the antigen-bearing target cells. (Some twenty lymphokines have been identified, although the specific functions of all of them are not known. One is interferon, an antiviral protein. Another is lymphotoxin, which is "poisonous" to the invading antigen. A third is MIF, for "migration inhibition factor," which apparently attempts to localize the reaction by drawing macrophages to the vicinity and keeping them there. Macrophages are large phagocytes, a word derived from the Greek and literally meaning "eating cells"; phagocytes are white cells that function more or less as cleanup crews, ingesting dead or incapacitated cells, including those of pathogenic organisms and other foreign material as well as worn-out cells discarded by the body itself in the normal course of events.)

The T cells also apparently function as "helpers" in the B cells' operations. And some daughter cells of both types are modified, coded or "programmed" to "remember" that antigen and to immediately respond in a similar manner upon subsequent encounter with it.

Inflammation is the visible evidence of this defensive process, whether it appears in the throat in response to a streptococcal infection, in the nose when tissues there are attacked by a virus, or in the skin surrounding a splinter. The immune system and its activities are necessary to life; were it not for them, we would succumb shortly after birth to the host of inimical agents and substances in our environment. Indeed, some children, victims of the uncommon congenital conditions called immune-deficiency diseases, are at just such risk and must receive regular injections of immunoglobulins or be kept in isolated, completely sterile environments. (There are several such conditions, of varying degree and severity. The most serious one follows a classic X-linked mode of inheritance and affects chiefly boys.)

The situation in lupus is precisely the reverse. Not a deficiency but a surfeit of immunoglobulins causes the problem. Further, the lupus patient's lymphocytes appear to act indiscriminately, staging attacks not only against foreign invaders but against her own tissues and organs. One might, in fact, describe their actions as deliberately discriminatory, singling out such tissues for their punishing activity. Why does this happen? Or, conversely, why *doesn't* it occur in the vast majority of individuals?

It must be emphasized at this point that the foregoing description of the immune-response process is based on observations to date—but that the entire area is under continuing investigation; very little was known or understood concerning these mechanisms until the past decade. What follows is in large part speculation.

To begin with, remember that the lymphocytes' actions

are initiated only by encounter with specific antigens. Normally, an individual's lymphocytes are evidently programmed to ignore the body's own antigens—cell-surface "flags" that communicate an "I belong here" message; only cells that do not belong, those with potential for compromising the integrity of the body, are singled out for destruction. The former kinds of cells are let alone, tolerated; the latter are not tolerated and are attacked.

Intolerance is another word for allergy. There are some substances that are inherently harmless to the human body and are so perceived by most of those bodies. When an individual exhibits an unusual inflammatory reaction to a substance—whether it be a pollen, a food, or a medication—we say that individual is allergic to that substance. As we have noted, lupus patients appear to have a heavier incidence of such allergies than other people. Typical of the investigations that have provided such data was one conducted at Johns Hopkins University in 1973; 26 percent of a group of lupus patients, versus 10 percent of a control group, reported a history of hives; 35 percent of the lupus group, but only 20 percent of the controls, reported a history of drug allergy (often in the lupus group, but not among the controls, manifested by arthritic symptoms). We don't know what this might imply.

And lupus patients appear to be, in a sense, also "allergic" to their own tissues.

A number of theories have been suggested to explain this anomaly.

One such theory, that of "sequestered antigens," postulates that some chemical substances occurring naturally

within the body may somehow be hidden away during
early embryonic development, while the lymphocyte-
producing organs are "learning" to recognize the individual's own cellular material and developing "tolerance" to
it. Later, when these substances are released into the circulation from wherever they have been sequestered, they
encounter mature lymphocytes which fail to recognize
them and thus behave exactly as if they were entirely foreign antigens. Since no one has demonstrated an antena-
tal cache of hidden antigens, this hypothesis does not appear to be the likely answer.

Another speculation, which might be called the "shot-
gun" theory, holds that the immune response in autoimmune disease might actually be directed at a truly foreign
antigen and that some of the body's own tissues fall victim as well. This theory might in fact explain rheumatic
fever, which has long been considered a hypersensitive or
"allergic" reaction to streptococcal infection; in more than
half of all rheumatic fever patients, there has been found
an antibody to streptococci that also reacts to myocardial
(heart-muscle) tissue (the condition is sometimes called
"autoimmune carditis").

The question of course arises as to why the defender
cells lack the ability to distinguish between the invader
and the native tissue; a heart-muscle cell is quite different
from a bacterium. One possible explanation is that the native tissue has been altered in some way, conceivably by a
bacterium, virus, or other pathogenic organism, so that its
antigenic identification is blurred; such a phenomenon,
involving a virus, has indeed been suggested in relation to
both multiple sclerosis and lupus (see Chapter 7).

If the native tissue has not been biochemically altered, then it must be assumed that something has gone awry in the immune-response process. (The two possibilities are not, of course, mutually exclusive.) Which brings us to the last part of our chapter title: the "forbidden clone."

Part of the initial immune reaction we described earlier consists of cloning—replication of a generation of identical daughter cells by a lymphocyte. It is possible that occasionally, in everyone, an aberrant lymphocyte arises, one that is capable of taking destructive action against that individual's own tissues. For the body's own health and survival, this is not a good thing. Therefore, it is postulated, there must be a built-in "control mechanism" that normally eliminates such randomly arising cells or inhibits their action, "precensors" them and prevents their generating a "forbidden clone," a group of cells capable of constitutional injury.

In lupus and other autoimmune disorders, the hypothesis goes, the self-protective mechanism fails to function: the randomly emerging, erroneously "keyed" lymphocyte, uncensored, does proceed to replicate, and produces what should not be: the forbidden clone. Those who have put forth this theory suggest that the renegade lymphocytes are B cells, and that the T cells may—in addition to acting as "helpers" and "instructors"—have a "suppressor" function that halts inappropriate B-cell behavior; the forbidden clone thus suggests T-cell deficiency. Since the forbidden clone is presumably generated in the same manner as an approved clone, there would also be daughter cells "memory"-coded to go into similar action every time the antigen is encountered—a frequent occurrence when the antigen in question is a part of the body itself.

A number of circumstances can be cited that fit rather neatly into the forbidden-clone scenario.

The thymus, the endocrine gland responsible for the T cells, is active in childhood but atrophies after the first couple of decades of life. (It will give you some idea of how knowledge of this subject has progressed if we tell you that until a very few years ago, the thymus had not even been classified as an endocrine gland and no one was sure that it had any function at all.) It also produces a substance, tentatively classed as a hormone, that has been named thymosin. While the relationship of this substance to T-cell maturation is unclear, thymosin has been extracted from calf thymus and used successfully to treat congenital lack of immunity associated with under-development of the gland, presumably based on a deficiency of "helper" T cells.

If thymus atrophy suggests that the T cells' "control" function is meant to decline with time (assuming there is such control in the first place), that would dovetail with the rarity of autoimmune disease in childhood. It would also explain why increased levels of gamma globulin can commonly be detected in most healthy individuals of advanced age.

While thymosin activity (which can be detected by certain tests) normally declines after the age of twenty or thirty—and is not detectable at all after the age of fifty—this process evidently takes place prematurely in lupus patients, as at least one small reported study has shown. Dr. Jean-François Bach of the Clinique Néphrologique in

Paris assayed thymosin activity in 22 lupus patients, all in the usual lupus-onset age range and some described as "very young." In 19 of those patients, he found *no* detectable thymosin activity *whatever*.

A particular set of animal experiments also bears out the forbidden-clone theory. There is a line of inbred chickens genetically susceptible to autoimmune thyroiditis (inflammation of the thyroid gland). It has been shown that the disease process in the fowl can be accelerated if the thymus gland is removed—and that the condition is ameliorated upon removal of the particular site in which the B-cells are known to mature in this species. It is clear in this instance, at least, that it is the B cells which perpetrate the damage and that the T cells (or the thymus gland itself, or both) have a controlling influence.

The fact that immunoglobulins are produced in excess in lupus similarly points to B-cell hyperactivity—and since a single lymphocyte is coded for a single immunoglobulin, the high levels during active inflammatory periods do, again, support the forbidden-clone hypothesis.

It has been suggested that drug-induced lupus—which, as we pointed out in Chapter 2, appears to be limited and not self-perpetuating—may result from a change in internal environment, effected by the drug, that permits forbidden-clone development. Withdrawal of the drug then presumably restores the status quo—suggesting either that the forbidden clone lacks "memory"-coded cells *or* that the drug somehow negates or inhibits T-cell "suppressor" activity and that normal T-cell activity resumes after a time if the offending drug is not reintroduced.

For the sake of completeness, we should mention that

another factor—or possibly two other factors—may also play a role. The reader may have read of a substance called *cyclic AMP*, isolated in the late 1950s; the letters stand for adenosine monophosphate, the "cyclic" being a description of its molecular structure. Its discoverer, Dr. Earl Sutherland, dubbed it a "second messenger," since it is active throughout the body and appears to "transmit" the "messages" of various hormones. It has also been demonstrated in the laboratory, though not in living beings, that cyclic AMP prevents the untoward proliferation of B lymphocytes.

It has been suggested that thymosin performs with the assistance of cyclic AMP and that thymosin may stimulate an enzyme called adenylate cyclase; the latter is known to trigger the production of AMP—which, in turn, may in some way work to increase the number of functional T cells.

There has since been isolated another substance, called cyclic GMP, which stands for guanosine monophosphate; this substance, it is postulated, acts in opposition to AMP. Like cyclic AMP, cyclic GMP is put into production by the action of an enzyme, here one called guanylate cyclase; the presence of calcium is necessary for that action and also for the maintenance of GMP levels.

Under normal conditions, these substances presumably keep each other in check, as do many opposite-acting substances and structures in the body, and help to maintain a balanced, or healthy, state. But an imbalance could conceivably occur. It is possible that a deficiency in adenylate cyclase—or excess levels of calcium, or of enzymes associated with GMP activity—might result in domination of the delicately balanced system by cyclic GMP. Theoretically, such a relative deficiency in cyclic AMP could lead directly to the unchecked proliferation of trouble-making B lymphocytes.

None of these suggestions precludes a possible role played by gonadal hormones, by genetic influences, or by pathogens such as viruses; it seems probable, in fact, that all the elements we have discussed in this chapter and the three preceding chapters interact in some way to produce the full-fledged disorder. That probability is strongly supported by research experience over the years with an animal strain that has provided a near-perfect laboratory "model" of lupus.

9. The Model Mice

Much of what medicine would like to know about lupus—or any malady, for that matter—is inaccessible. It's true that more and more sophisticated diagnostic and analytic techniques have revealed a wealth of information and that cautious use of new therapies has immeasurably improved the outlook for patients.

But there are potentially informative and/or beneficial techniques that simply would not be carried out on a human being, because they would be unthinkable. Human patients are not given massive doses of new drugs with totally unknown effects. They are not castrated or relieved of other glands or organs to observe the effects, if any, on their illness. They are not subjected to potentially lethal injections of pathogenic organisms or carcinogenic substances in order to challenge the competence of their immune systems. They are not executed at various ages and stages so that their organs might be laid out on an autopsy table.

These things *can* be done with laboratory animals. It is thus fortunate when a condition similar to a human ailment can be created in an experimental animal, providing a convenient subject for study and for therapeutic trials. Just such a situation has been extremely helpful, for example, in rheumatoid arthritis: inflammation experimentally induced in the joints of laboratory animals has resulted in much useful information, of direct benefit to arthritis patients, regarding the effects of rest, of physical stress, and of the administration of various anti-inflammatory drugs.

It is even more fortunate when a "model" is found—a particular animal that *naturally* develops a disorder paralleling a human ill. That fortuitous circumstance has occurred in lupus.

In 1959, it was reported by Drs. M. Bielchowsky, B. J. Helyer, and J. B. Howie that a strain of black mice native to New Zealand appeared to develop autoimmune hemolytic anemia spontaneously. This disorder, in which antibodies are formed against the individual's own red blood cells, also occurs in human lupus. Subsequent studies confirmed that the anemia afflicting the mice was also characterized by increased immunoglobulins, proteinuria, and nephritis involving the deposition of antigen-antibody complexes. All animals of this strain are subject to the disorder.

Genetic studies of that strain and others were begun.

Many hybrids were produced, displaying many variations of disease. Drs. Helyer and Howie soon determined that crossbreeding the New Zealand black (NZB) mice with a white (NZW) strain resulted in a hybrid that naturally developed an ailment even more striking in its resemblance to systemic lupus—and with invariable occurrence of the serious kidney damage that afflicts as many as half the victims of lupus.

Both the NZB mice and the NZB/NZW hybrids have since been under intensive study in laboratories around the world. The findings and observations that have thus far emerged bear uncanny resemblances to many of the data and theories detailed in the foregoing chapters.

The mice do not develop joint problems. Nor do they exhibit skin lesions—even if induction of such lesions is attempted by clipping or shaving their hair and exposing them to strong ultraviolet light for long periods. But other facets of their disorders are clearly relevant.

The NZB mice develop their disease by the age of twelve to fifteen months (the normal lifespan of an ordinary mouse is up to three years), although some become ill as early as three months of age. Antierythrocyte antibody is produced, and it is strictly a self-destructive agent: it will attack the erythrocytes of other mice (and of rats to a very slight degree) but not the blood of other animals or of humans. The result is a severe anemia that appears within weeks, with progressive weight loss. The anemia is most severe, curiously, in virgin females; in female mice that have been bred, it is statistically a little less severe than in males (although individual animals do show differences from these general pictures).

Some of the NZB mice prove to have antinuclear antibodies and some do not, but there are significantly increased levels of immunoglobulins, in particular IgG and IgM. There is also a high incidence of peptic ulcers (suggesting, possibly, antibody that reacts to the animals' intestinal mucosa), which afflict nearly every animal eventually if it lives beyond the age of two years.

In the NZB/NZW hybrids, it is severe kidney deterioration that predominates, and the damage seen is very much like that which can occur in lupus, primarily involving the glomeruli, the kidney's filtering units. The syndrome usually starts between the ages of three and six months (two to four months earlier in females than in males); it becomes in a few short weeks very much like a long-standing, particularly severe, and totally untreated case of human lupus. Titers of antinuclear antibodies rise quickly. The kidneys lose their function very rapidly: seven eighths of the mice die of uremia within six months —and since the disease process begins earlier in the females, their lives are cut even shorter.

Antibody against double-stranded RNA is found in a majority of the hybrids, as is antibody against DNA; the latter appears to parallel the severity of the renal disease and is present earlier and more often in the females than in the males. (A few of the males, for reasons unknown, seem to "stabilize"; although they eventually succumb to the disease, their condition remains at a chronic "plateau" for a time, rather than plunging downhill.) There are also an accompanying anemia and deficiencies, as in lupus, of the various types of blood cells. Many of the mice develop a disorder of the tear glands and salivary glands much like Sjögren's syndrome in humans.

All the factors cited in Chapters 5 through 8 as key clues to the cause of lupus are operative in the model mice as well.

As we've said, in both strains the females are the more severely afflicted. Whether the sex hormones play a part is still an open question. Dr. Norman Talal of the University of California at San Francisco has reported that if NZB males are castrated at the age of two weeks, their disease pattern tends to reflect that of the females—suggesting that the male hormones play a protective role. Spaying of female NZB mice results in decreased production of anti-RNA antibodies (although there is no effect on levels of antibodies against DNA). If the thymus gland of either sex is removed, the effects are those of gonad removal. Dr. Talal's conclusion: there is some action of the sex hormones on the thymus, that affects antibody production.

Some other investigators, however, have tried similar tactics in the NZB/NZW hybrids—castrating or spaying, and then administering hormones of the opposite sex—and have reported that in neither sex is the disease pattern modified in the direction of the other's.

There is absolutely no question, of course, about familial factors in the mice; their disorders are clearly congenital. It is also clear that transmission is genetic rather than transplacental: if fertilized ova from disease-free mice are transplanted to the uteruses of NZB mice for gestation, the offspring are perfectly healthy and do not develop any autoimmune disease.

The inheritance pattern appears dominant, since all the

mice of these strains are affected. It is not classically sex-linked; hybrids are affected whether the mother is NZB and the father NZW, or vice versa. There is, however, a somewhat different pattern of disease in these two situations: offspring survive longer when the mother is NZB and the father NZW than when the crossbreeding is reversed. Further, the differences affect offspring differently depending upon their sex. Male offspring of an NZB mother and NZW father survive an average 68 days longer than sons of an NZB father and NZW mother; some of the former have been known to live as long as thirty months. In females the average survival difference between the two types of parentage is only 20 days—which still represents a radically curtailed lifespan, since all female offspring of NZB fathers and NZW mothers are dead by the age of sixteen months. These differences remain unexplained.

It has, at any rate, become clear that the mode of inheritance follows no known classic pattern. The short lives of the model mice have permitted extensive crossbreeding among the two original strains and various hybrids; none of this has clarified matters. It is generally believed that whatever the pattern, several different genes are involved rather than a single one.

That there is a viral factor is also deemed highly probable. It has been demonstrated that there is at least one virus *associated* with the disorder, although a *causal* relationship has not been established.

There is a group of viruses, apparently distributed throughout the animal kingdom, that have been tentatively labeled "C types" because in some instances they are known to cause cancers. Such viruses have been identified in reptiles, birds, and several mammals including mice, cats, and monkeys. They are evidently species-specific, that is, each such virus has been isolated only from a single species of animal. They do not always cause malignant disease; in fact, they usually do not, and under normal circumstances their carcinogenic activity is apparently held in check by an automatic mechanism in the host.

Unlike other viruses, the C viruses are transmitted from parents to offspring and are thus present from birth. Antigens to such viruses have been found in the model mice by many investigators, and particles suggestive of such viruses have been found in their spleens, kidneys, livers, bone marrows, and a number of other organs. As in human lupus, there have been suggestions that antibodies initially aimed at the viruses are "misdirected" to attack native tissues as well, possibly because the latter have been altered in some way by the virus and release material perceived as a "foreign" antigen. It might be added that the malignancies known to be caused by C viruses are usually lymphomas, involving overproduction of lymphocytes by the spleen and lymph nodes.

Dr. Jay Levy and his colleagues at the University of California at San Francisco have shown that a specific C virus is transmitted—not only in the model mice but in all other strains of house mice they checked—within the egg and sperm cells, meaning that the viral genes must be incorporated with those of the host. This particular virus, interestingly, cannot infect mouse cells—but *can* infect cells of other animals. Dr. Levy calls the virus "xenotropic" ("foreign-material-attracted," from the Greek *xenos,* "stranger").

He theorizes, from the fact that the virus is found ubiquitously in mice (although the NZB strain has a bit more of it than others), that the virus is normally harmless and possibly even helpful at some stage of embryonic development. And that some genetic defect in the model mice gives rise to autoimmune disease—whether because inordinate quantities of virus stimulate antibody production or because in these mice the virus alters native cell antigens so that they are no longer recognized as "self."

Certainly, as in human lupus, there is some defect of the immune-defense system of these experimental animals —and again interest has focused on the distinct roles played by the two different types of lymphocytes, the B and T cells.

It has been shown by several investigators that there are such things, in the mice, as "suppressor" T cells (hypothesized in humans) that control B-cell activity and prevent overproduction by the latter of inappropriate immunoglobulins. This "suppressor" activity lessens in all mice as they age, and there is a small amount of autoimmune activity in elderly mice just as there is in elderly people. The model mice appear to reach this stage quite prematurely—and the autoimmune activity is of course not minimal but massive.

The proportions of the two types of cells in the blood, spleen, lymph nodes, etc., of the model mice are normal. But both the NZB mice and the hybrids display structural abnormalities in their thymus glands—which, the reader will recall, is where T cells mature. An NZB or

NZB/NZW thymus transplanted to a normal mouse (after removal of that mouse's own thymus) can actually induce autoimmune disease, proving that there is *something* about the abnormal gland that is involved in the etiology of the disorder.

High levels of immunoglobulins—which are elaborated by the B cells—are, as we mentioned earlier, found in the model mice. Deposits of immunoglobulins (especially IgG), described by investigators as "lumpy," have also been found in their damaged kidneys.

These extra immunoglobulins, however, do *not* confer extra resistance to attack by other organisms. The young model mice are capable of resisting such attack. But that capability diminishes rapidly, and it has severely deteriorated by the time the autoimmune disease has set in—a process demonstrated by viral challenge at various stages. It thus seems that in these animals a population of competent lymphocytes has been diverted from their normal defensive functions into full-time auto-antibody production.

In sum, the model mice appear to suffer from an immune system gone awry: inability to establish tolerance to their own tissues, permitting the emergence of "forbidden clones" that produce great quantities of self-destructive antibodies—coupled with simultaneous degeneration of normal, desirable immunocompetence. There are patently hereditary factors involved, whether or not the genetically transmitted virus plays a part. And the thymus gland is somehow associated with the disease process.

That last point has suggested a number of experiments.

Dr. Talal has, for example, tried injecting bovine thymosin into young NZB mice once a week. He found that onset of their disease was thereby delayed, but it was not prevented. And similar hormonal injections in older mice, in whom the disorder had already been established, had no effect whatever.

Dr. Alfred Steinberg of the National Institute of Arthritis, Metabolism, and Digestive Diseases, taking a slightly different tack, has tried injecting young NZB mice biweekly with thymus cells taken from newborn normal mice. His "patients" did not become ill until their injections were discontinued at the age of one year—while an untreated control group had all developed the expected anemia by the age of four or five months. He suggests that the injected material contained "suppressor" T cells, possibly releasing a "censor" substance that effectively prevents inappropriate antibody production.

That something in the normal mouse thymus is missing in the model mice is evident; it is not, however, merely a matter of the abnormal thymus producing the disorder. Thymectomy—complete removal of the thymus—has been performed on newborn mice of both strains; autoimmune disease is not prevented, and is in fact somewhat accelerated in the NZB/NZW hybrids. (If thymectomy is followed by a graft of normal newborn-mouse thymus, there is no effect one way or the other.) This acceleration of the disease process in the hybrids may suggest a partial protective role played by some component of NZW inheritance.

It appears that the spleen is a contributing factor in the disease: it is a busy center of antibody production as well as a site of erythrocyte (red-blood-cell) removal. Hence, another experimental surgical technique has been splenectomy. Results have been a bit puzzling. Young NZB mice thus treated have gone on to develop the disorder, but with less severe anemia and more severe renal disease than usual; yet, in older NZB mice, splenectomy has exacerbated the anemia and hastened death. Young NZB/NZW hybrids whose spleens are removed also become ill eventually, but their typical kidney disease is less severe than usual and they enjoy prolonged survival; the course of illness in older hybrids who are splenectomized, on the other hand, is not altered at all.

Since certain drugs are known to induce lupus in humans, a number of such drugs have been given to the model mice; they have included such frequently suspect substances as procainamide, hydralazine, and mesantoin. Effects: none whatever.

As to medications, concentration has narrowed down to much the same sorts of agents that have been found helpful or potentially helpful in human lupus, in particular the cortisone family and the immunosuppressants.

Corticosteroids, as in human lupus, have beneficial effects. While not curing the mouse disorders, they do control them, as evidenced by reduction in such gauges as proteinuria and antinuclear antibodies and in the severity of renal disease.

The immunosuppressant azathioprine has proved ineffective in one of the strains and hazardous to both. While it does not influence the course of the disease in the NZB mice, it does improve the kidney-disease picture in the NZB/NZW hybrids. But in both groups its use has been associated with an alarming incidence of thymus cancer; the precise reason is not known.

The most impressive therapeutic results in the mice have occurred with the immunosuppressant cyclophosphamide, particularly in the hybrids. Given to young mice, it appears to postpone development of the disease (but not prevent it) and prolong survival. In older mice with active kidney disease, there have even been full remissions—and in some instances actual healing of lesions. But, again, there is a hazard. While brief use of the drug appears safe, long-term administration has been associated with increased incidence of a variety of malignancies.

Presently, a number of investigators are looking into the possibility of multidrug therapy using corticosteroids and immunosuppressants in combination with each other and with other agents.

Two additional therapeutic avenues, on which initial reports were presented at a scientific conference of the American Rheumatism Association section of the Arthritis Foundation in December 1976, are also currently being pursued.

One of these involves the prostaglandins, a group of substances very much in the forefront of biomedical research. These substances—at least fifteen have been distinguished thus far—are synthesized in various tissues throughout the body and appear to act in conjunction with other substances, such as enzymes and hormones, to produce a variety of physiological effects, some of which are contradictory: while one may, for example, inhibit blood clotting, another may encourage it. Based on their chemical structure, the prostaglandins appear to fall into four groups, which have been designated by the letters A, B, E, and F and further differentiated by numbers; the Es and Fs appear to be most prevalent and active. The prostaglandin of special interest to lupus researchers is PGE_1—which had previously been found to stimulate the release of cyclic AMP (see Chapter 8) and also to reduce the joint inflammation of arthritis induced in laboratory animals. It now appears that injections of PGE_1 can dramatically prolong the lives of NZB/NZW mice, staving off the kidney inflammation that is the fatal factor in the hybrids' disease.

A second potentially fruitful path may be the use of antiviral agents. Several such experimental agents are being evaluated. One that appears to hold promise is called ribavirin; it seems to diminish inflammatory activity in the kidneys of the hybrid mice—as indicated by reduced proteinuria and antibody levels—and to prolong their lives by weeks or months.

And research into the patterns and possible causes of the mouse disorders of course continues. Many perplexing questions remain.

Why does autoimmune disease inevitably afflict each generation of mice, yet, in defiance of Darwinian principle, permit the apparently genetically flawed strain to survive? What is the mechanism of hereditary transmission? How significant is the relative severity of anemia in the virgin NZB females—and the severity of disease in the female mice generally? Do hormones produced by the male mice play a protective role, albeit an incomplete one? Is there, despite conflicting research results, a potential therapeutic role for such hormones? Where does the thymus gland fit into the picture? Why do thymus transplant and the injection of thymus cells have such different effects? How can the contradictory results of splenectomy in the two experimental strains be explained? What roles are played in the mouse disorders by viruses or other environmental factors?

The answers to these questions may well point the way to the long-sought solution to the puzzle of lupus itself.

INDEX

Acetaminophen, 38–39
Acetyl transferase, 64–65
ACTH (adrenocorticotrophic hormone), 42
Age of lupus patients, 55
Aldomet, 15
Alka-Seltzer, 39
Allergy in lupus patients, 18–19, 35–36, 39–40, 87
American Rheumatism Association (ARA), 19–23, 25, 62, 105
Androgens, 56, 62
Anemia, 11, 22, 45; in drug-induced lupus, 16; in experimental mice, 95, 96
Animal studies, 91, 94–107
Antibiotics, 45; and drug-induced lupus, 15–16
Antibodies, 24–26, 83. See also Antigen-antibody reactions; Antinuclear antibodies; B cells; Immunoglobulins
Anticonvulsants and drug-induced lupus, 16
Antigen-antibody reactions, 8, 24, 28–29, 43, 85–93, 100
Antihypertensives and drug-induced lupus, 15
Anti-inflammatories, 38–40
Antimalarials, 36–38
Antinuclear antibodies (ANA), 24–26, 62, 63, 75; in experimental mice, 97
Anxiety, 34
Apresoline, 15
Aralen, 37–38
Arthritis associated with lupus, 10, 13, 21, 31, 34n, 38. See also Rheumatoid arthritis
Arthritis Foundation, 34n, 105

Aspirin, 38–39
Atabrine, 37–38
Autoimmunity, 9, 83–93; in experimental mice, 96, 101
Avascular necrosis, 46
Azathioprine, 43–44, 104–5
Azolid, 40

Bach, Jean-François, 90
B cells, 84, 85, 89–92, 101–2
Bielchowsky, M., 95
Blood casts, 21
Blood-cell deficits, 22
Blood pressure, 41, 45
Blood tests, 21, 22–29; false-positive for VD, 11, 13, 21, 62
BUN (blood urea nitrogen), 47–48
Butazones, 40
"Butterfly" rash, 6, 20

Calcium, 92–93
California, University of, 98, 100
Cama, 39
Camoquin, 37–38
Carbamazepine, 16
Cardiac involvement, 14, 16
Celontin, 16
Chicago, University of, 25
Chloroquines, 36–38
Chlorpromazine, 15
Christian, Charles, 81
Circulatory disorders, 46. See also Blood pressure; Lipids
Clinique Néphrologique (Paris) 90
Cold, 35
Collagen diseases, 7–8
Complement, 28–29

T4